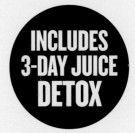

INCLUDES
3-DAY JUICE
DETOX

Keeping it Simple!

Juice Master

OVER 100 DELICIOUS JUICES & SMOOTHIES

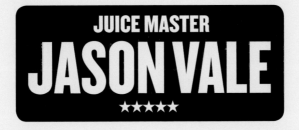

JUICE MASTER

JASON VALE

★★★★★

HARPER
thorsons

HarperThorsons
An imprint of HarperCollins*Publishers*
77–85 Fulham Palace Road,
Hammersmith, London W6 8JB

The website address is: www.thorsonselement.com

H A R P E R
thorsons

and *HarperThorsons* are trademarks
of HarperCollins*Publishers* Ltd

First published by HarperThorsons 2007

15 14 13 12

A catalogue record of this book is available
from the British Library

ISBN 978-0-00-722517-0

Printed and bound by Printing Express
Hong Kong

NB While the author of this book has made every effort to ensure that the information
contained in this book is as accurate and up-to-date as possible at the time of publication,
medical and pharmaceutical knowledge is constantly changing and the application of it to particular circumstances depends on many factors. This book should not be used as an
alternative to specialist medical advice and it is recommended that readers always consult
a qualified medical professional for individual advice before following any new diet or health programme. The author and publishers cannot be held responsible for any errors and omissions that
may be found in the text, or any actions that may be taken by a reader, as a result of any reliance
on the information contained in the text, which are taken entirely at the reader's own risk.

Contents

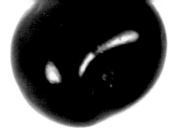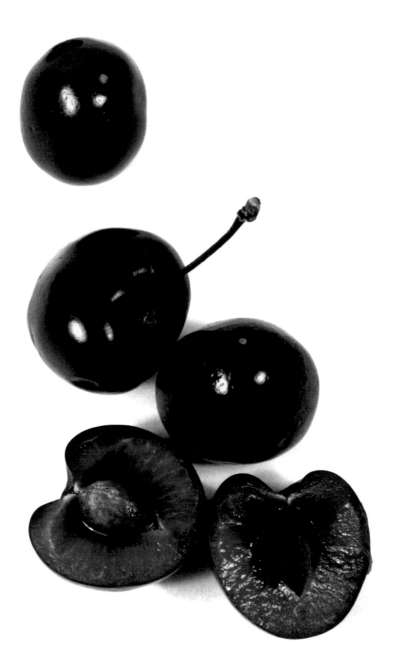

Not Simply Another Juice Recipe Book!

What you are holding is **not** simply another juice recipe book. In fact, if you're looking for something which goes beyond the usual, 'here's a bunch of recipes, now get on with it' type of juice book – then you are holding it.

Yes, there are recipes – over 100 tantalizing, melt-in-the-mouth, let your taste buds dance for joy recipes – but there are also many inspirational juicy extras. Juicy extras that will take this book from one which simply snugs in between Jamie, Nigella and Gordon not doing very much – to a book that you will actually use on a regular basis.

It seems crazy that as a nation we buy more recipe books than any other country in Europe, yet we also buy twice as many take-aways. The average person will make a maximum of just four recipes from a recipe book; the majority of people make just ONE!

My aim is a simple one – to get you truly inspired so that you will make as many of the mouthwatering recipes in this book as possible. The title of this book is Keeping it Simple and one thing I have learnt more than any other over the last juicy decade is that juicing needs to be made super-simple and super-fast in order for people to truly embrace it into their lives. I have also learnt that just a little bit of extra juicy knowledge can make all the difference between a book that has one recipe made from it and one that has loads of juicy stains because it is used that much.

Recipes to Sejuice You

If I said to you that you should juice two apples and a third of a lemon with the skin on as it makes a nice tasting juice which is good for you, you may or may not be tempted. However, if I said that by juicing two crisp Golden Delicious apples and a juicy wax-free lemon you would produce a rich, creamy, frothy juice which tastes **identical** to sherbet lemonade, but without any artificial anything, the chances are you would be more inspired to make it. If I then added that this simple yet incredibly delicious combination contained vitamins A, B1, B2, B6, and C, beta-carotene, calcium, iron, magnesium, phosphorus, potassium, sulphur, amino acids, anti-oxidants, natural sugars, pectin and boron, the chances are you would be even more likely to want to make it. If I then added that this combination helps to cleanse the liver and kidneys, flush the body of excess toxins, sweep the intestines, is excellent for the skin, hair and nails and helps to build immunity to common ailments − the chances are you would be getting your juicer out before I had a chance to finish the sentence.

Not Just About the Drink

This is what makes this juice recipe book so different from most of the others. Not only have the recipes been extremely well thought out and taste simply divine, but each one has a list of all the vitamins, minerals and other nutrients they contain along with exactly how each juice or smoothie will benefit you.

There's the Juice Master's Natural Pharmacy, where you will find juices for specific ailments; the Kids' Stuff section about how to get kids to 'drink their fruit 'n' veg', if they aren't eating it; No Sweat recipes designed for the athletes amongst you and even a Sexy Juice section, containing recipes to help lift your energies in the bedroom! And there's so much, much more.

However, before you get your juicer out and start sampling some of the simply gorgeous juices and smoothies, I feel it's always best to get a full understanding of …

The Power of Raw Juice

I have been extremely privileged to bring a juicy lifestyle to hundreds of thousands of people all over the world. When I set out to 'Juice The World' I never truly envisaged the incredible impact juicing would have, not only on virtually every aspect of physical health, but also on people's mental well-being and life in general. A recent study has shown that simply drinking fruit and vegetable juice three times a week reduces the risk of getting Alzheimer's disease by 76 per cent, so imagine the difference juicing makes to general mental sharpness. This is just one of literally thousands of studies which have looked at the effects that juicing has on our mental and physical health. Over the years, studies have shown that virtually every ailment known to wo/mankind has either been completely alleviated by drinking freshly extracted raw fruit and vegetable juices or reduced dramatically – including the big 'C' (cancer).

However, as impressive as some of these studies are, what I find far more powerful are the stories which come directly from people who have incorporated juicing into their daily lifestyles. There are stories of incredible permanent weight loss; hair changing back from grey to black; stories of skin conditions clearing completely; of energy levels exploding.

I know first hand the sheer power of the juice. I suffered from severe asthma (I used an asthma inhaler 14–16 times a day), incredibly bad psoriasis, eczema, hay fever and one of the most common ailments to hit the UK population – being overweight. I know what it feels like not only to suffer from these conditions but also to be told by a doctor that there is no cure for some of them at all. Yet by simply swapping my normal junk(ie) foods and drinks for a freshly extracted juice or two a day and by adding a touch of exercise to daily life, my mental and physical health improved beyond anything I could have envisaged. My asthma is now just a memory (and I was told there was nothing I could do about it); my psoriasis has cleared by 90 per cent (I was literally covered from head to toe in this extremely challenging skin disorder and I was again also told it is a condition where 'diet plays no part'); my eczema has vanished; and I am no longer overweight. I didn't take any pills, creams or potions and yet miraculously my symptoms either drastically reduced or disappeared altogether.

Creating Pure Magic

We should never underestimate the power of **freshly extracted** fruit and vegetable juices. Each glass is a far cry from 'just a nice drink'. Every time you extract the vitamin- and mineral-rich juice from the fibres of fruits and vegetables you have pro**juiced** something medical science can but only dream of replicating. While they can isolate and name some of the vitamins and minerals contained within the juice, there is no way they can possibly manufacture anything which can come close to it. Nature has the true X factor and we will never truly know exactly what elements go into the liquid fuel contained within all fruits and vegetables. This liquid fuel has the power to furnish the system with vitamins, minerals, natural sugars, natural fats, amino acids, anti-oxidants, enzymes and organic water. This liquid fuel is designed to carry life-giving nutrients to exactly where they are required whilst at the same time flushing the system of any rubbish which may have accumulated.

When you make a juice I want you to understand fully that you aren't simply making a rich, creamy, better-tasting version of something you can otherwise buy in a bottle from the shops. I want you to understand fully that when you make a **freshly extracted** juice of any kind, you are creating magic. Magic may seem like an over-the-top word to use when all we appear to be talking about is a 'juice'. However, there is simply no other word that can sum up the life- and health-changing effects of freshly extracted juice. Skin begins to glow, hair starts to shine, nails get harder, eyes become brighter, excess fat appears to just melt away and ailments which have been disabling for years just vanish. David Copperfield managed to create the illusion of making the Statue of Liberty disappear, but that's about all it was — an illusion. The magic that happens when you pour fresh juice into your bloodstream on a daily basis is very real. After all, giving the impression that the Statue of Liberty has vanished is one thing, but having the power to make something as life-debilitating as asthma disappear is nothing short of pure magic.

Magic Doesn't Come in a Bottle

This 'juice' magic only occurs with **freshly extracted** juice. Please never be deluded into thinking that any juice or smoothie you buy in a shop comes anywhere close to what you can make fresh at home. What most people aren't aware of is that ALL shop bought juices and smoothies (even the innocent-looking ones which are 100 per cent 'natural') have been 'heat-treated' or pasteurized — a process which destroys a large section of vitamins, minerals and all enzyme activity (the life force of the plant). The only way to get the full taste, nutritional benefits and that bit of pure juicy magic is either to get one from a **good** juice bar or make one yourself at home.

Most juice bar smoothies are made with **pasteurized** juice and often have sugar-loaded yogurt. Believe it or not but when you see a juice bar shouting about their 98 per cent fat-free yogurt, you are usually getting yogurt loaded with sugar. The base juice they use is nearly always from either concentrate juice or pasteurized juice. They then put a fresh banana in and you think it's all totally live and fresh. It amazes me when I see big chain juice bars declaring: 'The only sugar found in our juices are those from nature'. This sounds all well and good, but they are talking about the small selection of juices they have —

not their smoothies. So, as you can see, the **only** way to get some real juice magic is to either find a extremely good fresh genuine juice bar (see the list at www.juicemaster.com) or get your juicer out and make your own.

Creating Theatre

Making your own juice ensures you know exactly what went into it, how clean and fresh the produce is and whether it's genuinely organic or not, and it also gives you the chance to create some theatre at home. That is what I love the most about juicing and smoothie making – it creates atmosphere and theatre in the kitchen. Kids are mesmerized by juicing. Seeing all the vibrant colours of fresh fruits and veg being juiced and blended before your very eyes and hearing the blender in action is a much more vibrant way to start your day than with a bowl of sugar with milk over it!

Just seeing juice coming out of a seemingly solid object (like a pear) is amazing in itself. But once you start not only to taste the difference of fresh juice compared to the bottle stuff, but also – and more importantly – feel and see the results, your juicer will play as big a part in your life as your kettle.

Replenishing Your Health Bank Account

None of us are perfect on the food and drink front, but one thing is for sure, every time you pour the liquid fuel contained within the fruits and vegetables into your body, you are replenishing your enzyme ('life') bank account. This is probably the most important account you will ever hold and it's worth knowing that when you eat and drink the wrong things, you are effectively dipping into this precious account. The 'life' bank manager often sends 'warning statements' to say you are slowly but surely using up your account and at this rate the account may be closed much earlier than expected. These 'warning statements' come in the form of headaches, weight gain, skin disorders, arthritis, etc. We often ignore such warnings and just carry on as normal, popping a few aspirin along the way (the equivalent of tearing up the statement and putting it in the bin). This is one account you really don't want to overspend on – once it is spent, so are you!

By simply having even just one **freshly extracted** fruit/veggie combo juice a day, you are doing more to top up your life account than the average Briton does in a whole week (we haven't just been voted 'The Fattest Nation In Europe' for nothing!).

So **before** the 'bank manager comes knocking' GET JUICED! There is a quote I used in one of my previous books, Turbo Charge Your Life In 14 Days, which sums up the importance of keeping ourselves healthy. It came from an 87-year-old man who, when asked what his secret was -- he looked much younger, had all his own hair (not a grey one in sight), all his own teeth and was fit as a fiddle – he replied that he never ate junk food. When they asked 'but why' (as in 'life is too short'), he simply replied: 'The reason I don't eat junk food is because unless I look after my body I'll have nowhere to live.' The biggest irony is that this 87-year-old man lived on the streets and got all his fresh produce from the local market – the guys down there gave him a load at the end of each day.

So, unless you look after your body you will have nowhere to live – somewhere to survive perhaps, but nowhere to truly live. The good news is, no matter how much you have dipped into your life account, it's never too late to top it up. The even better news is that no matter how many years you have been withdrawing, the minute you start to replenish it, it starts showing on your account extremely quickly. Make a point of having a fresh juice a day and the compound interest will bring you health benefits which are nothing short of magical.

The Right Juicy Kit

There is nothing more important to living a juicy lifestyle than getting the right juicer. Let's be real, juicing has been seen as a bit of a pain in the proverbial for years. The shopping and chopping of the fruit and veg were always seen as a juicing bugbear, but the biggest juice 'put me off' by a mile was always the cleaning.

The good news is that juice extractors have come a long way in the last few years, and technology has now made carrying heavy fruit and veg a breeze; one click of a mouse and a couple of bags of nature's finest can be at your door within the hour.

When I first started juicing I could never understand why they didn't make a wide chute so that fruits like apples could go in whole. It seemed like a no-brainer to me, yet all the juicers that were on the market when I started had very tiny chutes. This always meant spending an enormous amount of time cutting up the produce for it to fit into the feeder. Not only that, but all the juicers had small 'pulp containers', which meant that after making just one or two small glasses you would have to stop the machine, take it apart and put it back together before continuing. Worst of all, though, was the cleaning. There were so many parts to the average juicer, so many nooks and crannies where the pulp could get caught up in and the machines were so small and fiddly that it just took forever to clean them properly. The words 'dishwasher safe' were never found on a juicer as the plastic parts would warp and melt from the heat of the washer.

Despite all of that, the benefits of juicing far outweighed the hassle of making the juice and cleaning the machine — but I did long for the day where juicing would become easy.

21st–century Juicing

Luckily, that day has arrived. Twenty-first-century juicing is here and with it comes wide-chute juicers, more extraction, large pulp containers for continuous juicing **and** dishwasher safe machines! Even as I write there are even efforts underway to produce a self-cleaning juicer. Imagine that, a juicer that cleans itself automatically after you make a juice. OK, stop dreaming, that day isn't here yet, but the day of super-fast juicing is. In fact, with some of the best models on the market today you can make juice for four people **and** quickly clean the machine in less than 10 minutes. Even though many machines are now dishwasher safe, there are so few parts to them that it's almost as fast to clean them as it is to rinse them ready for the dishwasher.

Get the right juicer … for you!

Getting the right juicer is crucial to whether juicing makes a regular appearance in your life, or whether the machine stays in your cupboard for good! It is extremely important to get the right juicer for your needs. For our purposes, up until now, there have been just two basic types of juicer:

Masticating (slow juicers) Centrifugal (fast juicers)

They both have their pros and cons. The main difference is that 'slow' juicers tend to live by their name: they are slow to use, slow to clean and tend to cost more; however, the **quality** of the juice tends to be superior. Whereas 'fast' juicers are exactly that: fast to use, fast to clean and tend to be cheaper than masticating juicers. The problem with fast juicers is about the **quality** of the juice: Most have powerful motors that cause the cutting blades to move at incredibly high speeds in order to juice super-fast. This creates 'heat friction' and heat affects nutrients. It is well documented that the longer you cook something, the more nutrients you lose. This means the juice oxidises and separates much faster than with a slow juicer and tends to be of inferior quality in comparison. This doesn't mean the juice from fast juicers is void of nutrients; you are just encouraged to drink the juice as soon as possible after making it. The best fast juicers on the market as I write this page are the Philips range of juicers.

The Game Changer In The Juicing World!

Up until now these have been the main choices of juicer to get. Both are really good and I have been recommending a *whole fruit* fast juicer for the past ten years and I have also talked about the virtues of slow juicing. The vast majority of people choose a fast juicer because of time restraints, but ideally want the quality of a slow juicer. The good news is that every now and then a game changer comes into the market. The iPod did it, and so did companies like Dyson; they completely changed the game in their field and I am pleased to say we have a game changer in the juicing world too. It's a juicer that's almost combines the best of both worlds in juicing: 'slow' and 'fast'.

The Fusion of Technologies

From now on when people ask what juicer you have, it will be a case of 'fast, slow or FUSION'. The Fusion Juicer is just that: a fusion of both juicing worlds. You can fit a whole apple in it like a fast juicer, but the low-induction motor means it extracts the juice without anywhere near as much heat friction. This means the quality of the juice is comparable to an expensive slow juicer. It's also easy to clean (everything goes in the dishwasher), it's whisper quiet, it looks good and it's VERY affordable. My mission since I started on my own health journey has been to JUICE THE WORLD and one of the most important aspects of making sure that mission is achieved is to a get a juicer into every household in the world. That can only happen if the juicer is incredible value and affordable by all. But usually the best value juicers aren't the best juicers, and I have, until now, always recommended more expensive juicers. The Fusion Juicer is not quite as fast as a super-fast juicer and not quite the quality of a £400 slow juicer, but it's a beautiful combination of the two. With the Fusion you get a juicer that doesn't heat the juice like a fast juicer but is a million times faster to use than a slow juicer. You get a juicer that produces the highest-quality juice but for a quarter of the price and from a machine that's easy to clean. You also get a juicer where you can see the juice being made in the juicer itself. This creates theatre in the kitchen and kids love to see the colours going round.

Personally, if I were getting into juicing for the first time or looking to change my juicer, the Fusion Juicer would be my only choice. I am not the only one who is excited about this juicer: Jon Gabriel, a remarkable man who lost over 200lbs (91kg) with the help of juicing and raw food said "I have been waiting for this juicer for years. Finally, a juicer that is fast to use but doesn't create massive heat friction". I said it was a game changer and it is.

Having said that, new juicers are coming out all the time and by the time you read this particular version of this book things might have changed, so before buying any juicer please always visit www.juicemaster.com and see what's new in the juicing world!

Hey Big Blender!

The other piece of kit you will need for your juicy kitchen is a blender or a 'smoothie maker'. Not all blenders can the job, so look for one that can also crush ice, blend soft and frozen fruits and demolish an avocado. There are some blenders which claim to be juicers, like the excellent Vitamix blender; but it's still a blender. A juicer juices and a blender simply blends the fibres with the juice. You need both for a juicy lifestyle.

Do The 3-Day Super Juice Detox

I have included a 3-Day Super Juice Detox in the book and if you wish to see the positive effects of juicing in a short space of time, I strongly advocate doing it. Not only will you drop an average of 3-5lbs on the program (some people when adding exercise drop 7lbs in just 3 days), but it also gives the digestive system a much-needed rest from dealing with the processed rubbish we pour into it on a weekly, if not daily basis.

Since the first edition of this book I have made one tiny adjustment to the original 3-Day Super Juice Detox program, by adding more avocados. This slight addition has made no difference to the positive effects on both a mental and physical level and more importantly for many, the weight loss is exactly the same, despite adding in an extra 3 whole avocados over the 3 days. This surprises some as a medium avocado has around 250 calories. However, despite what you may have heard from mainstream dieticians, calories aren't all the same. What the addition of avocado has done however is to increase the success rate of people who start and complete the program. Many who tried the old version of the 3-day juice plan said they found doing my 7lbs in 7 Days Super Juice Diet easier than the 3-day detox.

When I looked at the plan again I could see why some might find it a little challenging. As it was a 3-day plan and not a 7-day plan, I wanted people to have maximum weight loss results, so I left out avocado for the most part, having just two in the 3 days. The absence of enough avocado meant some found themselves incredibly hungry on day one and so some threw in the towel. The good fat and amino acid content of avocados helps to regulate the appetite. The old version also had the addition of my Detox Booster powder, which, while adding some great nutrients to the plan, wasn't to everyone's taste. Just because you are on a Detox, it doesn't mean it has to feel like you are. And so to some, with hunger hitting and taste marred by the Detox Powder, it felt like a detox! The 'new and improved' 3-Day Super Juice Detox removal of the DETOX BOOST powder (you can still add if you want to and don't mind the taste), and the addition of more avocados. This may seem like an inconsequential change, but with the addition of a decent amount of avocado in the first two smoothies of the plan, it makes it a great deal easier as you wont be hungry. The shopping list for the program can be found on www.juicemaster.com and is free to download. We also have a 3-day wall planner to make it even easier and also an iphone App. By doing the 3-Day Super Juice Detox you will get used to using your juicer and blender, you'll get the hang of cleaning it and you will reap the weight loss and health rewards, all of which will give you the incentive to make juicing part of your daily life.

Juice The World!

One mission has driven me more than any other for many years now and that is to 'Juice The World'. My aim is to make a juice extractor as common as a kettle and toaster in every home in the developed world. I genuinely believe that a juice extractor is one of, if not the, most valuable purchase you will ever make. It is the ultimate health insurance aid and no home should be without one. Every week at Juicy HQ we receive emails, cards and calls from just about every corner of the globe saying how juicing has changed their lives in one way or another. Whether it's healthy weight loss, an improved illness, increased energy or just that their eyes have began to sparkle again and their skin is as clear as a whistle. Just read Audrey's email on the next page …

Whatever it is I never tire of hearing how juicing has had a positive effect on someone's health and it is one of the many things, find juicing has a positive effect on your life, or anyone you know, please drop us a quick note at info@juicemaster.com, I sincerely hope you make juicing part of your daily life and I may get to meet you personally at one of my juicing retreats in the future. At time of writing I have just bought a little retreat in Portugal, which I am turning, into Juicy Oasis – Health Retreat & Spa. It's in the middle of nowhere and every room overlooks the magnificent lake. Maybe I'll see you there for a juice and game of tennis one day, if not I hope juicing benefits your world as much as it has mine.

Enjoy the book!

the recipes

kids' stuff

if you can't get your kids to eat it — get them to drink it!

Let's face facts: on the whole most kids just hate eating veg. They don't mind a bit of fruit from time to time, but sit them down to some raw broccoli and they're more likely to stick it in some soil and shout 'bonsai' than actually eat the stuff! However, turn it into nature's finest liquid fuel, mix it with, say, some fresh pineapple or apple juice, and bingo — they're licking their lips in seconds.

Kids are mesmerized by juicing. When they see fresh juice coming out of a solid vegetable like a carrot, they're transfixed. Little Molly, my two-year-old friend who pops round most mornings for her morning juice, loves veggie juice. Yes, you heard it right, a two-year-old who drinks vegetable juice! Not only does she drink ingredients such as beetroot, celery, cucumber and carrot, but she even makes the juice herself (with supervision, of course!). She's not the only one either. I now know hundreds of kids, from age two upwards, who are consuming the finest body and brain builders known to wo/man on a regular basis. In fact, juicing and smoothie making is simply the best way of getting raw live fuel into your kids without the usual nightmare of trying to get them to eat it.

Juicy kids tip

Get your little 'bin lids' to brush their teeth after their juice or swill some water around their mouth. Even good sugars can be harmful to growing teeth! Come to think of it, adult juicers should do the same.

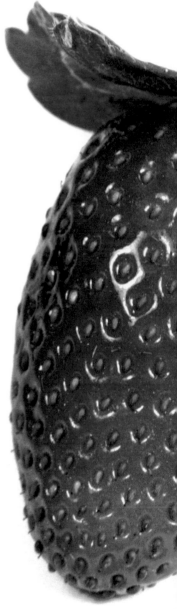

popeye power

Freshly extracted apple, pineapple, spinach and lemon juice over ice

With 'Popeye' in the title there are no prizes for guessing one of the main ingredients in this recipe. Spinach isn't usually top of the list when it comes to kids' favourite foods and if they see you putting the green stuff into this recipe you may have a fight on your hands trying to get them to drink it. This is why sometimes a little white lie can be a good thing. The juice is really green and if you tell them it's kiwi fruit that has made it that colour and that it's a fruit juice, your chances of getting them to drink it will improve massively. Having said that, some kids don't mind the fact it has some spinach in (like little Molly – she even puts it in the juicer herself!), but only you know your child and if you need to tell a slight porky on this occasion, it's not a bad thing.

1 large handful **spinach**
¼ medium **pineapple** (peeled)
1 **apple**
1 inch slice **lemon** (unwaxed if possible, if not peel it)
ice

Juice everything and add ice. Remember to pack the spinach into the feeder of the chute before turning on the machine and then push it through slowly. If you have a whole fruit juicer, place the apple in first, then the spinach, then the pineapple and lemon.

Look what's in it! Vitamins A, B1, B2, B3, B6, C and E, beta-carotene, iron, magnesium, potassium, calcium, chlorophyll, sulphur, bioflavonoids, folic acid and natural sugars.

How will it juice the little ones? Helps to maintain healthy skin, eyes and bones. This juice is good for boosting the immune system, great for cardiovascular health and the niacin (vitamin B3) is an excellent aid for brain and nerve function. Although spinach is well known for its iron content, not all is in a form easily utilized by the body; however, much more becomes available in spinach juice. And, with pineapple containing iron too, the Popeye certainly contains more than enough for your little ones' needs. Very cleansing.

kids' fruity special

Freshly extracted orange, apple and kiwi juice, blended with banana and ice

We all know fruit is good for the kids, but very few realize just how good. You may think a carton of fruit smoothie is a healthy alternative to a refined white sugary drink, and you would be right, but few understand the power of a freshly made fruit smoothie. A smoothie that hasn't been heat treated; a smoothie that has nothing but fresh, live ingredients. Very few have any concept of the quantity of vitamins, minerals and anti-oxidants that nature provides in every fruit on Earth. Make a smoothie for your kids and you will not only be giving them a delicious drink, but a great deal of what they need to grow both physically and mentally.

1 juicy **orange** (peeled, but leave the white pith on)
1 **apple** (Golden Delicious or Royal Gala)
¼ **banana** (fairtrade if possible)
1 **kiwi fruit** (green or gold)
ice

Juice the orange, apple and kiwi. You can juice the kiwi fruit with the skin on, but this can often be harsh on the back of the throat, so it's your call on that one. Place the banana in the blender, along with the juice and ice. Blend until smooth.

Look what's in it! Vitamins A, B1, B2, B6, C and E, beta-carotene, fibre, magnesium, potassium, folic acid, boron, ellagic acid, amino acids and natural sugars.

How will it juice the little ones? Kiwi fruit are rich in beta-carotene, which is converted into vitamin A when the body needs it. This vitamin is essential for the development and growth of cells and helps maintain healthy skin and eyes. Vitamin B1 (found in apples) assists in blood formation and the production of hydrochloric acid, which is essential for proper digestion. Fibre helps to keep kids 'moving' and the potassium to keep their sodium/ potassium balance in order (perhaps after they have eaten too many crisps!).

Juicy tip

If you tell your kids exactly how smoothies will help them, they are much more likely to ask for them. If we are dealing with teenagers, it's good to mention that they 'help to keep a good healthy weight' and are 'great for clear skin' — you know the things they worry about.

kids' chute juice

The idea of the book is 'Keeping it Simple' and a whole fruit juicer makes juicing that much easier (see The Right Juicy Kit, page 9). Kids' Chute Juice has been designed with whole fruit juicing in mind. All of the ingredients fit into the chute, you push down and boom — juice done! If you don't have a wide funnel juicer, you can clearly still make this juice; it just means you have to spend some extra time cutting, chopping and feeding into the chute. This gorgeous-tasting fruit smoothie packs more nutrients than you would think. Just look at what's in it below to see the incredible quantity of vitamins and minerals your kids will get by having a small glass.

2 **apples** (Golden Delicious or Royal Gala)
⅓ **lemon** with rind on (unwaxed if possible)
1 **pear** (Conference are best, but use whatever you can get hold of)
ice

Put one apple in the chute, followed by the lemon and pear. Sandwich with the other apple and juice. Add ice to cool.

Look what's in it! Vitamins A, B and C, potassium, folic acid, boron, ellagic acid, carotenes, amino acids, natural sugars and anti-oxidants.

How will it juice the little ones? Pear juice is exceptionally good for protecting the colon. Given that colon cancer is now one of the biggest killers in the UK, the earlier you can get some protection into your kids the better. The mineral boron is needed in trace amounts for healthy bones and muscle growth. It is also necessary for the metabolism of calcium, phosphorus and magnesium. Additionally, it enhances brain function as well as playing a role in how the body utilizes energy from fats and sugars. Both apples and pears contain boron.

choctastic

It may come as a surprise that chocolate has made it into a recipe for the little ones, but the only chocolate used here is over 80 per cent cocoa. It is also organic and fairtrade (the most important aspect). The incredible amount of goodness found in the combination of fresh banana, orange, pineapple and live yogurt more than quash any negative effect the chocolate may have, and if it's the only way the little chaps will consume fruit then it's all for the greater good.

1 **orange** (peeled, but leave on the white pith)
1 inch thick slice of a medium **pineapple**
4 pieces organic **chocolate** (use fairtrade, above 80 per cent cocoa solids)
½ **banana** (fairtrade if possible)
3 tablespoons low-fat live **yogurt**
ice

Juice the orange and pineapple. Grate chocolate into the blender (mind your fingers!) and add banana, yogurt, juice and ice. Blend everything until smooth – soooooooooo tasty!

Look what's in it! Friendly bacteria, calcium, vitamins A, B6 and C, sodium, potassium, magnesium, iron, folic acid, phosphorus, zinc, beta-carotene, fibre, natural sugars, amino acids and anti-oxidants.

How will it juice the little ones? Live yogurt helps replenish the friendly bacteria in the gut, helping to prevent any overgrowth of yeast. Calcium helps neutralize an acidic system and is, of course, good for the bones and teeth. The juice contains nature's natural balance of sodium and potassium, one the key factors to good health, and even the dark chocolate contains some anti-oxidants. This is an extremely balanced smoothie that tastes naughty but is still extremely good for your kids.

kids' stuff

reddy, steady, go!

Freshly extracted apple, beetroot, broccoli, celery, cucumber, pineapple and lime juice

Raw beetroot is not on top of most kids' wish lists on the food front, but it is unbelievably good for them. Once again, this is where juicing comes into its own. When you juice raw beetroot it gives a gorgeous deep red colour and the taste is surprisingly sweet. It's not one you would drink on its own, but mixed with a few other veg and a serving of fruit, you can fool any kid into believing that they are having a nice berry juice! Reddy, Steady, Go! is a wonderful recipe, full of veg, yet it tastes like fruit — a parent's dream. Designed to get the kids 'ready' for anything; to have a 'steady' supply of nature's fuel going into their systems and to give them that juice 'go'.

2 **apples** (Golden Delicious or Royal Gala)
1 small raw **beetroot**
1 small **broccoli** stem
½ **celery** stick
1 inch slice **cucumber**
½ inch slice **pineapple** (diced to fit into feeder)
1 **lime** (peeled)
ice

Put one apple in the chute followed by the beetroot, broccoli, celery, cucumber, pineapple, lime and then 'sandwich' with the other apple. Juice the lot, then add ice to cool. All juices taste better when cool, especially veggie ones!

Juicy Note: You can juice pineapple with the skin on, it just depends if your juicer can take it. Oh, and don't forget to wash it well.

Look what's in it! Vitamins A, B1, B2, B3, B5, B6, C and E, iron, calcium, sodium, manganese, chlorine, bioflavonoids, potassium, folic acid, boron, ellagic acid, carotenes, amino acids, natural sugars and anti-oxidants.

How will it juice the little ones? Beetroot is one of nature's finest blood builders. The nutrients in this juice are good for young brain function, great for their growing bones, extremely hydrating (an excellent natural diuretic); they are also antibacterial, help with constipation, and are excellent for nails, hair and skin. This is an all-round amazing juice.

Juicy Note: If your kids' 'poo' turns red, don't panic – it's the beetroot. (Of course, if this should continue, see your GP.)

> **'** I have been overweight all my life, constantly trying to slim down. Since reading your book, I've lost weight and never been happier or felt better. **,**

Jenny

kids' stuff

so berry good

Freshly extracted pineapple juice, natural live yogurt, fresh blue and blackberries

Of all the recipes in this 'Kids' Stuff' section, children love this one more than any other. The good news is that it is not only incredibly sweet and delicious, but also one of the healthiest smoothies you can make. If you are at all concerned about your kids' health, pour one of these in a flask and stick it in their packed lunch every day.

¼ medium **pineapple** (fairtrade wherever possible)
1 handful **blackberries**
1 handful **blueberries**
100g low-fat live **yogurt** (if vegan, this can be left out)
4 **ice** cubes

Juice the pineapple and place all other ingredients in the blender — blend until smooth.

Look what's in it! Vitamins B1, B2, B6, C, E, all the essential amino acids, natural sugars, essential fatty acids, good bacteria, anti-oxidants, calcium, iron, magnesium, phosphorus, sodium, zinc, folic acid, bromeline, potassium and ellagic acid.

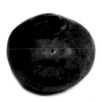

Why is it sooooooooooooo berry good for the little chaps?

It is so good that if I wrote everything this wonder smoothie could do, it would take a mini-book in itself. It's packed with anti-oxidants, which help to keep your kids' skin as soft and clear as the day they were born. So Berry Good is also packed with anti-ageing vitamin E and amino acids — the building blocks for the entire body. If you thought it couldn't get any better, this super smoothie is even loaded with essential fatty acids, vital for heart protection and good elasticity in the skin and is a rich source of calcium and iron. This really is one of the most powerful smoothies you will ever make your kids — and they'll love it!

Juicy boost

For extra acai and goji berry goodness, add 1 heaped teaspoon of Juice Master's Ultimate Berry Boost. These two anti-oxidant stars are the new super-foods on the block and make this berry good smoothie super berry good!

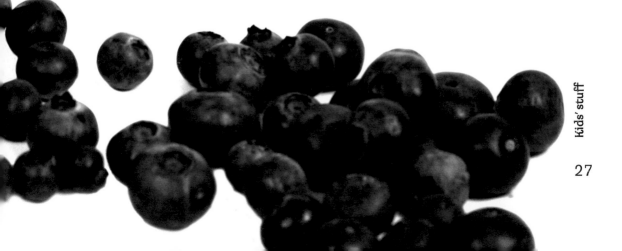

kids' stuff

27

juicy schools

I love speaking at schools. My whole juicing philosophy of 'if you can't eat it – drink it' is never more apt than when teaching kids healthy eating (or drinking, to be more accurate in this case). On one occasion I had to leave Cornwall at 2am in order to drive to a school in Ramsgate for 8.30am. I remember having only 1–2 hours' sleep (if that) and thinking on the way: 'Why did I agree to do this again?' However, the second I started the talk and saw the transfixed looks on so many willing-to-learn kids' faces, I knew why I had made the long journey. They were astonished by juicing and smoothie-making and they all had a go at making juice and tasting even the most vegetable of juices. Much to their, and the teacher's, surprise, they loved them!

At the end of the session I threw open a competition. Whoever came up with the best recipe would get into my new book. Out of all the recipes I received this one stood out, for the way it was written more than anything else. It also tastes damn good.

'Thank you for your talk. You really made me think. I approved of the vegetable juice that you served. I could see what you meant by the 'earthy' taste, but other than that, I thought it did taste like 'liquid sunshine'. I also learned that a fruit smoothie is a perfect thing to wake up to in the morning. Thank you again for your talk.'

Jack

my fruit and vegetable smoothie

(by Paris Duce, year 5)

½ **lemon**
1 **apple**
½ **orange**
1 handful of **grapes**
1 handful of **raspberries**
4 **strawberries**
½ **cucumber**

Juice the apple, orange and lemon and add to the blender with all the other ingredients. Blend until smooth.

"I just want to say your recommendation of the juicer was excellent because it does its job brilliantly. I love orange juice and crapple [a mixture of carrot and apple juice]. I enjoyed your book thoroughly. I was wondering if you could recommend a juice or a smoothie I could have when I come back from school as a snack."

Johnny

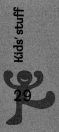

detox

the body does indeed clean itself naturally — but only if it is given the chance to do so!

'Detox' is a bit of a buzz word in the world of health and nutrition, but not everyone buys into it. Many people, particularly in the medical world, often dismiss the notion that we ever need to detox. They reason that the body naturally 'detoxes' all the time, regardless of what we do.

This is true, the body does indeed clean itself naturally — but only if it is given the chance to do so! If you constantly pollute the environment in which your cells bathe there will always be a degree of toxicity in your system. There isn't a wild animal on the planet who ever needs to 'detox', but, then, there isn't a wild animal on the planet who pollutes their system either.

This is why it is so worthwhile to give your organs and digestive system a much needed rest from the burden of all that processed food. It just so happens that a juicy detox is a wonderful way to do it. To get you started here's my 3-Day Super Juice Detox, but all of the following recipes can be used for a 1, 2, or 3-day detox.

Juicy boost

To fast-tox your detox, simply add a teaspoon of Juice Master's Ultimate Detox Boost powder (see page 13) to any of the detox recipes.

Juice Master's 3-Day Super Juice Detox

Enlightenment in Just 3 Days!

I am aware that the above headline sounds like one of those suspect flyers that come through the door and I am more than aware that mentioning getting lighter as a benefit of this Super Juice Detox programme could be seen as just a tad shallow (OK, very shallow). However, I am also aware that as much as we may hate ourselves for it, 'shallow' tends to beat health when it comes to reasons for going on a detox of any nature. Tell someone their system will be cleaner after a juice detox, they might decide to go on it. Tell them their stomach will be flatter and BOOM — they're on it faster than high speed broadband.

Personally I am not bothered what the incentive is that gets people juicing, I just want them to experience it and make it part of their **daily** routine. If you are attracted to a flatter stomach and that's what gets your juices flowing, then cool. If you are driven more by the health benefits, then again — fantastic.

> ❛ I have just finished the 3-Day Super Juice Detox and I must write to thank you. I have lost 5 pounds in just 3 days and have experienced 'enlightenment' (love that expression). Moreover I just feel so much better. I did experience some 'detox' symptoms, as you mentioned I might, but it was nothing and certainly worth it for the way I feel now. Thank you again for making juicing part of my daily life. ❜
>
> Anna

If you are overweight then clearly I am not suggesting you will get a flat stomach in just 3 days, but it will certainly **feel** and **be** much flatter than it was before you started. However, the best effect of this 3-Day Super Juice Detox is how it affects your mental state. Once you clean your system of caffeine, refined sugar, refined fats and other junk for 72 hours and flush and nurture your body with the finest freshly extracted 'live' fruit and vegetable juices, your nervous system becomes calmer, you start to think clearer and you begin to notice a heightened mental sharpness and awareness. The beautiful knock-on effect is that as your system becomes more 'alkaline' and you start to feel physically and mentally lighter, cravings for junk are reduced and the desire to eat and drink well are increased. This is why it is very rare for anyone to simply do a detox of this nature and go back to exactly what they were eating and drinking before they started. When you start to feel light, on both a mental and physical level, you create momentum and a desire to want to experience more of the same.

> ❛I have lost 5lb on your 3-day detox programme! Moreover I have a great deal more clarity. My mind feels lighter and I'm not as 'on edge'. The recipes are extremely well thought out and the information you give about every recipe is very useful. When I bought the book I expected a few good recipes and some juicing tips, but I got so much more. I will continue to juice daily - many thanks again Jason for a wonderful book. ❜
>
> Kate

Keeping Detox Simple

All you need to complete this programme is your juicer/blender, a flask, the appropriate fruit and veggies and, of course, the right attitude.

Juicy Detox Preparation

It's always good to be a little prepared for any sort of programme, but as you will be living on nothing but the finest juices and smoothies for 3 days, good preparation is of paramount importance. With that in mind, and with simplicity as our theme, here are your …

Detox

Top Ten 'Keeping it Simple' Tips for Your 3-Day Juicy Journey to Enlightenment

1. Be Prepared

You will find the programme so much simpler if you are fully prepared. Make sure you get all the fruit and veg you need (see 'Detox Shopping List' page 38) **before** you start. To make life easier, you can download the 3-day detox free of charge from www.juicemaster.com.

2. Make Sure Your Fridge is Empty!

This isn't always easy to do if you have a large family, but what I mean is, don't let any food go to waste. It is important that if you are starting on, say, a Monday, you don't then shop 'normally' two days before. If you do, what inevitably happens is that you start to think, 'I would do it now but all this food will go to waste', and you never get around to it. Let your food run down, **then** shop for the programme.

3. Get Mentally Prepared

Getting all the fruit and veg for this programme in advance is important, but even more so is the right frame of mind before you start. If you are familiar with my books you will know that I am huge on mental preparation. I was amazed to read one of the reviews on Amazon, referring to the 7lbs in 7days Super Juice Programme, saying, 'the first part of the book is pointless, but the programme is very good'. This may be true for some — after all, not everyone needs motivating and some are quite happy to get themselves into the right frame of mind — but for the vast majority a bit of mental encouragement is of paramount importance. Sadly, I don't have any room in this juicy recipe book to add some powerful mental juice. However, I would suggest you make a point of reading 'The Power of Raw Juice' (page 3). Once you read just how powerful a juice detox can be and the results you get on both a mental and physical level, you will be more than inspired not only to start the 3-Day Super Detox: Juicy Journey to Enlightenment, but actually complete it (what a concept!).

4. Get the Right Juicy Kit

The difference between a small-chute juicer and a wide-chute juicer is often the difference between success and failure. I don't simply mean success and failure with this detox programme; I mean it's the difference between whether you will juice for life or juice for a just a day! You may think that there's not a great deal of difference between having to cut an apple into four pieces and putting one in whole, but it's like night and day when you are making several juices a day. (See 'The Right Juicy Kit', page 8 – it will save you time, money and your sanity!)

5. Get The App!

If you want to make life easier for yourself, get the 'Juice Master 3 Day Detox' app for iPhone or Android. I have recorded coaching videos for each day to help guide you through any detox symptoms you may be having. It also has all the videos of how to make them along with a neat interactive shopping list. It's like having me in your pocket … you make your mind up if that's a good or bad thing!

6. Get a GOOD Flask

A flask will be an invaluable item, not only for this 3-day detox programme but also for your juicy life in general. In order to keep the vitamins, minerals, enzymes and so on at their best you really need to block out as much oxygen and sunlight as possible. A flask is the best way to do this and to keep your

Detox

juice as fresh as possible when on the go. Not all flasks are built the same and I highly recommend flasks made by the company SIGG™. We do our own Juice Master SIGG™ bottle on our website, but you can buy regular SIGG™ bottles in many places (and, no, I don't get royalties from them). Unlike most flasks, those from SIGG™ are moulded from one piece of metal and so don't have the tainted smell and taste that can sometimes occur with standard flasks.

7. Clear Your Evening Diary

You don't have to live like a hermit while on this programme, but as this is your juicy journey to enlightenment, it would be advisable to clear your evening diary to give your mind as much rest as your body. The programme is also much easier if you aren't being goaded by friends when out in a bar!

8. Turn Off The TV!

Can you go 3 days with no TV? You may say 'yes, no problem', but it's not as easy for everyone. The 3-day journey to enlightenment is not only designed to detox your body, but also your mind. TV is one of the biggest mind polluters in our modern world and several studies have been done which clearly show that you not only burn less calories when watching TV (than even doing nothing at all – yes, it's true!) but people tend to think about food much more when mesmerized by the 'life in a box'. Personally, I love a bit of TV as much as the next person, but a true journey to enlightenment can only happen when your mind is as clear as your body. While this is up to you, swapping TV for a book for 3 days will make a large difference to how you feel at the end of the programme.

9. SLEEP, SLEEP and SLEEP!

We live in a strange time in human development; it seems it is now almost a crime to admit you're tired. Whenever I'm tired the general response from people is: 'you can't be – you're the Juice Master!' Rest is as important as clean air, exercise, good nutrition and an attitude of gratitude, so please allow yourself to go with it (if you can!) over the next 3 days. You will find that when you stop putting false stimulants in your body such as caffeine, refined sugar, artificial sweeteners and so on, your body will naturally need plenty of rest to recover.

If you find yourself getting more tired than usual over the first couple of days, don't fight it – grab as much rest as possible and if you feel tired at 8pm – sleep! Your body will repair and detox much faster when you are asleep. This is why after a Saturday night out on the town, eating and drinking till the early hours, you wake up on Sunday with your mouth feeling like a sandpit, sleep in your eyes and a head like death itself. This is your body in 'detox' and 'clean' mode. You may well spend many hours awake and not feel a desperate need to shower, but after a night's sleep you are literally itching to have one. Allow yourself as much sleep as your life and people around you will allow!

10. Pamper Yourself

If you are going to do a detox then really do it. Your Juicy Journey to Enlightenment will be greatly enhanced with a little, or a lot, of pampering. I have got together with some gorgeous spas in the UK and abroad that offer my 3-day detox as part of a package. This is taking 'Keeping it Simple' to the next level. Simply lie back, have all your juices made for you, have a massage or two, perhaps a few gentle yoga sessions, relax in a hot tub, maybe a steam room, and be pampered – heaven! (For details of which spas offer the programme see www.juicemaster.com or call us on 08451 302 829).

Detox

Detox Shopping List

3 **Carrots**
22 **Apples** (not Granny Smith or Cox)
3 **Lemons** (unwaxed)
1 Yellow bell **pepper**
1½ **Cucumber**
3 **Celery** sticks
3 **Broccoli** stems (1 inch each)
1 large or 2 small **Beetroot** (raw)
2 pieces **Ginger** (fresh)
small handful **Parsley**
2 **Avocado** (ripe)
¼ cup **Blackberries** (fresh or frozen)
¼ cup **Blueberries** (fresh or frozen)
1 medium **Pineapple**
1lb (½ kilo) **Spinach**
3½ litres **Mineral water**

Detox boost

To fast-tox your detox, simply add a teaspoon of Juice Master's Ultimate Detox Boost powder (see page 13) to any of the detox recipes. Please note that by adding the powder you will change the taste. The powder is not essential and I would always try one first before adding to every juice.

The Programme

DAY ONE

On waking	Hot water with slice of lemon
Breakfast	Detox Special (page 40)
Lunch	Detox Special (page 40)
Linner	H_2O Detox (page 43) (Between **Lunch** and **Dinner** – **Linner!**)
Evening 'meal'	Beyond Detox (page 46)

DAY TWO

On waking	Hot water with slice of lemon
Breakfast	Super Detox Smoothie (page 44)
Lunch	Dreamy Detox (page 42)
Linner	H_2O Detox (page 43)
Evening 'meal'	Beyond Detox (page 46)

DAY THREE

On waking	Hot water with slice of lemon or lime
Breakfast	Detox Special (page 40)
Mid-morning	H_2O Detox (page 43)
Lunch	Beyond Detox (page 46)
Linner	H_2O Detox (page 43)
Evening 'meal'	Dreamy Detox (page 42)

juice master's detox special

Freshly extracted apple, carrot, lemon, pepper, cucumber, celery, broccoli and beetroot juice blended with ice

One of the main juices on the 3-Day Juicy Journey To Enlightenment, the Detox Special is packed with the finest green, yellow and orange juices, all of which are designed to furnish the system with optimum nutrition without putting a burden on the digestive system. This allows the system to detox naturally whilst giving the right nutrients and anti-oxidants to maximize the process of detoxification.

3 **apples** (Golden Delicious or Royal Gala)
1 **carrot** (organic if possible)
1 slice **lemon** with rind on (unwaxed where possible)
¼ yellow bell **pepper**
1 inch slice **cucumber**
¼ piece **celery**
1 inch **broccoli** stem
1 inch slice raw **beetroot**
1 medium or large ripe **avocado** (your call!)
ice

Place one whole apple in the juicer and then add all other ingredients except the avocado, finishing off with the final apples and juice. Place a couple of ice cubes in the blender along with the flesh from the avocado. Add the juice and blend until creamy and smooth.

Look what's in it! Vitamins A, B1, B2, B3, B5, B6, C, E and K, calcium, iron, magnesium, potassium, pectin, boron, ellagic acid, beta-carotene, folic acid, phosphorus, selenium, riboflavin and anti-cancer phytonutrients. Also contains amino acids (the building blocks for protein), essential fatty acids and a good source of carbohydrates.

How will this help to detox? Avocados provide nearly 20 essential nutrients, including fiber, potassium, Vitamin E, B-vitamins and folic acid. They also contain about 250 calories, which when on this juice only plan, you will be very grateful for. The good fat also helps to regulate the appetite. Celery helps to flush the body of excessive carbon dioxide and reduce acidity in the system. The beetroot is extremely good for cleaning the bloodstream and is excellent, along with lemon, for cleansing the liver and kidneys. Beetroot is also one of nature's finest blood builders. The high levels of beta-carotene in this juice help mop up harmful free radicals and strengthen the immune system.

dreamy detox

2 **apples** (Golden Delicious or Royal Gala)
1 slice **lemon** with rind on (unwaxed where possible)
1 inch slice **cucumber**
1 stick **celery**
1 inch piece fresh **ginger**
ice

Juice everything and place ice and juice in the blender. Blend until smooth. Remember that you can skip the blender if you wish and just add ice, but it's better and smoother with the blender.

Look what's in it! Vitamins A, B1, B2, B3, B5, B6, C, E and K, copper, calcium, iron, magnesium, potassium, boron, ellagic acid, beta-carotene, folic acid, phosphorus, selenium, riboflavin and anti-cancer phytonutrients.

How will this help to detox? Apple and cucumber are amazing for flushing out and cleaning the system. The celery helps to flush the body of excess carbon dioxide and reduce acidity in the body. Ginger is a well-known natural antibiotic and superb decongestant. Lemon is particularly powerful at removing harmful bacteria and toxins from the intestinal tract and is also amazing at cleaning the liver and kidneys.

Juicy Note: This recipe is in our Juice 'n' Smoothie bars up and down the country. Check out www.juicemaster.com to find your nearest Juice Master Juice 'n' Smoothie bar.

h$_2$o detox

This recipe can be used at any time, whether you are on the 3-day detox or not. It is particularly good for a 24-hour super detox. This is where you simply drink hot water with lemon, mineral water, this H$_2$O Detox and nothing else. This flushes the system and gives a full 24-hour break from any kind of heavy digestion. Lighter than a juice, but more filling than water.

1 inch piece raw **beetroot**
½ **apple** (Golden Delicious or Royal Gala are best)
1 inch slice **pineapple**
1 inch slice **lemon** with rind (if not unwaxed remove rind)
¾ litre mineral **water** (or your choice of water)
1 sports **bottle** or **flask**

Juice the beetroot, apple, pineapple and lemon. Mix with water into a large bottle (a 1-litre bottle should be big enough). Shake and drink (that's shake the bottle, not yourself!).

Look what's in it! Vitamins A, B and C, potassium, boron, carotenes, folic acid, manganese, calcium and iron.

How will this help to detox? This light juicy water helps to flush the system of impurities while supplying the body with essential nutrients. Beetroot is nature's best blood builder, the lemon cleans the liver and kidneys. Apple is nature's best-known detoxifier.

Juicy Note: This drink is also excellent for pre- and post-workout as it's rich in potassium.

Detox

43

super detox smoothie

Fresh **blueberries**, **blackberries** and low-fat live **yogurt** all blended together with **freshly** extracted **pineapple** juice and **ice**

Blueberries make a wonderful-tasting smoothie, but add some gorgeous whole blackberries, fresh pineapple juice and natural yogurt, and you have one of the most filling and nutritious smoothies in the book. This tasty smoothie will be a godsend if you are on the 3-day detox plan – the veggie stuff is great but you can't beat a fruit and yogurt smoothie thrown in every now and then to keep you sane!

½ small **pineapple**
1 handful fresh **blueberries**
1 handful fresh **blackberries**
200g low-fat live **yogurt** (or soya yogurt or soya milk)
4 **ice** cubes

Juice the pineapple and pour into the blender along with the blueberries, blackberries, yogurt and ice. Blend until smooth.

Super Simple Version of this Recipe You can make this recipe without a juicer if in a real hurry. You simply leave out the pineapple and place everything in the blender and blend until smooth. If too thick, add water or some soya milk.

Look what's in it! Vitamins B1, B2, B6, C and E, fibre, potassium, iron, calcium, manganese, beta-carotene, phosphorus, folic acid, anti-oxidants, zinc and sodium.

How will this help to detox? Blueberries contain some of nature's most powerful anti-oxidants and anti-ageing phytonutrients, which help to destroy the free radicals that age the skin and cause premature wrinkles. Blackberries are antibacterial, they promote healing and are also good for the treatment and prevention of diarrhoea. The live yogurt helps to maintain a healthy gut.

❛I read your book front to back and couldn't put it down because I was that keen to start! In 6 weeks I have lost almost 28lbs and it prompted me to get my life into gear. At 32, I have never felt or looked better. Thank you for helping me get my life sorted! ❜

Kay

beyond detox

Freshly extracted apple, spinach, beetroot, cucumber and parsley juice blended with avocado and ice

Beyond Detox has all the vitamins, minerals and anti-oxidants you would expect in a full-on detox.

3 apples
1 large handful **spinach**
1 inch raw **beetroot**
1 inch slice **cucumber**
Parsley (just a small amount – it's quite a powerful herb. Leave out if you have kidney problems or are pregnant)
½ ripe **avocado**
ice

Before turning on your machine, place one whole apple into your whole fruit juicer, then push down and pack the spinach and parsley tight before adding the cucumber, beetroot and other apples. If there isn't enough room for the other apples, simple follow through with them afterwards. Place the avocado into the blender along with the juice and ice. Blend until smooth – drink slowly and brush your teeth afterwards!

Look what's in it! Vitamins A, B1, B2, B3, B5, B6, B12, C, E and K, beta-carotene, calcium, iron, magnesium, phosphorus, sulphur, silicon, chlorophyll, folic acid, alpha-carotene, anti-oxidants, boron and amino acids.

How will this help to detox? Parsley is one of nature's superherbs. It expels worms, relieves gas, freshens breath, stimulates normal activity of the digestive system and helps bladder, kidney, liver, lung, stomach and thyroid function. Not bad for a little herb (pronounced ErrrB in the US!). This gorgeous smoothie contains all eight essential amino acids – the building blocks for protein. Every cell in your body and mind will benefit from it.

Juicy boost

To take this detox juice way beyond a simple detox, add 1 teaspoonful each of Juice Master's Ultimate Detox Boost and Juice Master's Ultimate Juice Boost. Their super-high concentration of vitamins, minerals, anti-oxidants, amino acids and chlorophyll transform 'beyond detox' into a 'wonder detox'.

the juicy pharmacy

'Let juice be thy medicine and medicine be thy juice.' Hippocrates said something similar

I'm not a doctor and don't claim to be. I don't have any sort of Dr title either. You know the thing. Some nutritionist or 'life coach' gets on a plane to the US, buys a Doctorate and shoves Dr in front of their surname in a bid to add a little cred to what they are saying. No, I am not a doctor and I don't have letters before or after my name. What I do have is over a decade's worth of juicing and nutrition experience and I've helped hundreds of thousands of people from all around the world with just about every common ailment known to wo/man. Also, I don't feel the need to look at your poo before seeing what you clearly need on a nutritional front!

When it comes to health I believe there are times when short-term, and even long-term, medical intervention is necessary, but I am much more sided with an 'alternative' approach. It seems somewhat nuts that 'drugs' are seen as the normal approach and every other approach is deemed 'alternative'. Personally I think of drug medicine as the 'alternative' approach — the alternative approach to what nature has to offer. I am a big advocate of nature's ability to nurture and treat every disease known to us today. Nature's high water content, vitamin- and mineral-rich foods and plants were designed as our best food source and our finest source of medicine. (Never underestimate the power of an apple or a lemon.) We have discovered very little of what actually makes up nature's superfoods, but one thing is for sure, if you stop eating and drinking rubbish and start to drink a few glasses of nature's live liquid fuel, amazing things will start to happen to body and mind.

I tend to shy away from the 'one juice for one ill' type of approach to health. The main reason for this is that the body works as one and so any freshly extracted juice will benefit the overall health of the system and help build the immune system. However, there is no question that certain fruits, vegetables and herbs can be of more therapeutic value than others when trying to treat a specific ailment.

With this in mind I have come up with 'The Juicy Pharmacy'. In this juicy section you will find not only some of the most therapeutic juices to be found on the planet, but also some of the tastiest. No more will you need 'a spoonful of sugar' to make this delicious medicine go down. If you are taking medication for any ailment please always speak with your GP or medical practitioner before either reducing or coming off the medication completely. Remember, I don't know your history and I am not a doctor. Equally though, if you feel you are starting to get better from whatever ailment, don't just continue to take the drugs blindly. Many doctors are enlightened these days and if they feel you are ready to start to come off the drugs, then they will tell you so.

recovery angel
the hangover helper

Mixed berries, fresh banana, low-fat live yogurt, fresh OJ ... and a little stroke of the head

A little worse for wear? Too much of the amber nectar? Feeling like your head is about to explode? Never fear, Recovery Angel to the rescue! This hangover helper is one of our most popular smoothies at our Juice Master Juice 'n' Smoothie bars, so if you are out and about or too hungover to actually make it yourself, come and see us and we'll make you one!

1 large **orange** (peeled but keep the pith on)
1 large handful **mixed berries** – **strawberries, blackberries, blueberries, raspberries** (in season fresh is best but you can get good quality frozen mixed berries from any supermarket)
1 **banana** (fairtrade where possible)
100g low-fat live **yogurt**
4 **ice** cubes

Juice the orange and pour into the blender. Add all other ingredients and blend until smooth. If you wish to make this in super-fast time you can get some fresh non-concentrate orange juice and pour into the blender with the other ingredients – this saves cleaning the juicer!

Look what's in it! Vitamins A, B6 and C, calcium, folic acid, iron, potassium, thiamine, magnesium, fibre, friendly bacteria, natural sugars, anti-oxidants, amino acids and beta-carotene.

How will it help my throbbing head and aching bod?

The oranges are rich in vitamin C, folic acid and an array of minerals, such as potassium – all of which are depleted by heavy drinking. The natural bacteria help replenish healthy bacteria in the gut, quelling any nausea or an upset stomach. The natural sugars help to raise depleted blood sugar levels and the organic water flowing through nature's finest fruits will re-hydrate your system.

Juicy Note: When you feel your head pounding after a night on the drink, most of what you are feeling is blood trying to pump through a dehydrated brain – nice!

migraine miracle

Freshly extracted **apple**, lemon, ginger, **spinach**, broccoli and **cucumber** juice all **mixed** together and **poured** over **ice**

I used to suffer from migraines and they aren't a good thing to have. All you can do is shut yourself in a very dark room, cut off all light and sound, and pray it goes away. Migraines are not headaches, they are a world apart, and my heart goes out to all those who suffer from them. However, the good news is that a study published in the *Lancet* magazine established that 93 per cent of long-term sufferers can obtain relief by eliminating certain offending foods; most common of these are cheese, chocolate, red wine, wheat, corn, eggs, milk, shellfish, citrus fruits, coffee and tomatoes. If you eliminate those foods and get this juice down you a few times a week, all should be well.

2 **apples** (Golden Delicious or Royal Gala)
1 large handful **spinach**
1 inch stem **broccoli**
1 inch slice **cucumber**
1 inch slice **lemon**
½ inch fresh **ginger**
ice

Place one apple in your whole fruit juicer and pack in the spinach. Then add the cucumber, lemon, ginger and broccoli and top with the last apple. Juice the lot and pour into the glass over ice.

Look what's in it! Vitamins A, B, C and E, potassium, pectin, boron, ellagic acid, carotenes, folic acid, iron, chlorophyll, magnesium, natural sugars, amino acids and anti-oxidants.

How will it help smooth away my migraine? The magnesium in lemon and green leafy veg is of great help to those who have hyperglycaemia. Studies have shown that people who suffer from migraines also tend to suffer from hyperglycaemia. The hydrating effects of freshly extracted juice helps blood circulation and the vitamin E in this juice has been shown to protect against some 80 diseases.

❛ I haven't had a migraine since I started juicing!
I experimented and for a week I didn't juice or exercise
(Pilates) and guess what — yes my migraines came back
with a vengeance! From the time I was a toddler I suffered
from migraines, at least once a month and sometimes twice
and three times. I have been to several doctors, clinics, done
the programme, took the pills for 30 years and nothing
worked. So thank you, Jason. ❜

Penelope

cold war

Freshly extracted **orange, pineapple** and **lemon** juice, blended with **ice** and sweet **Manuka** active **honey**

While it appears that there is no cure for the common cold, there is no question that a little rest along with the right juicy nutrients can certainly go a long way to help. This gorgeous combination of vitamin C and potassium, along with the active ingredients of the unique Manuka active honey, and the array of vitamins, minerals and anti-oxidants in the fruit, is the perfect combination to help stop the sniffles and get you back on your feet.

¼ **pineapple** (fairtrade if you can)
1 **orange** (peeled but leave the pith on)
1 inch of **lemon** (with skin on if unwaxed)
1 teaspoon **Manuka active honey**
4 **ice** cubes

Juice the pineapple, orange and lemon. Pour the juice into the blender and add honey and ice. Blend until smooth.

Look what's in it! Vitamins B6 and C, calcium, folic acid, iron, potassium, magnesium, beta-carotene, natural sugars, plus active antibacterial honey.

How will it help ward off my cold? This juice is loaded with vitamin C, which is not only a natural antibiotic but also helps dissolve mucus. The active Manuka honey also has powerful antibacterial properties. The impressive showing of the anti-cancer king – beta-carotene – and the enormous quantity of anti-oxidants all help to build your natural defences.

Juicy boost

For a super health injection, add a teaspoon of Juice Master's Ultimate Juice Boost before blending.

memory aid

Fresh **strawberries, raspberries**, low-fat live **yogurt** all blended together, freshly extracted **apple** juice and a little drop of **Ginkgo Biloba**

A study in the US released in 2006 which followed 2,000 people over a period of 10 years, showed that people who drank fruit and vegetable juice more than three times a week were 76 per cent less likely to develop Alzheimer's disease. If it can prevent a disease as extreme as Alzheimer's, imagine what it can do for day-to-day memory. As all juices can help, I have isolated a couple of ingredients that have minerals that are known to help memory.

2 **apples** (Golden Delicious or Royal Gala)
1 handful mixed fresh **raspberries** and **strawberries**
100g low-fat live **yogurt**
A few drops of **Ginkgo Biloba** (available in any good health shop)
4 **ice** cubes

Juice the apples and pour into blender. Add the raspberries, strawberries, yogurt, ice and Ginkgo biloba. Blend until smooth.

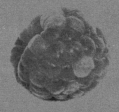

Look what's in it! Vitamins A, B, B1, B2, B6, C and E, ellagic acid, folic acid, beta-carotene, potassium, iron, niacin, fibre, friendly bacteria, zinc, calcium, phosphorus, malic acid, pectin, sulphur, anti-oxidants, natural sugars, amino acids and nature's Ginkgo X Factor.

How will it help my memory? A lack of zinc has been linked with bad memory; this is why I have included strawberries and raspberries, which contain high levels of zinc. Research on Ginkgo biloba shows that small doses can help cognition (aspects of understanding) and improve attention, information processing and short-term memory. Both healthy volunteers and people with mild memory problems were improved with ginkgo.

clear skin elixir

Freshly extracted **apple** juice, **spinach**, celery and **cucumber** juice all blended with **ice**

Having had both psoriasis and eczema I am more than aware of the discomfort and depression any kind of skin disorder can bring. I am also aware that by now you are probably fed up with everyone and their mother telling you what is best for it. Let me be clear here: one juice of anything, no matter what, will not cure you of eczema, psoriasis, or any other skin disorder for that matter. However, creating a more alkaline environment in your body and getting your essential supplements will go a long way to helping you. I still get the odd bout of psoriasis, but I used to be covered from head to toe 24/7 and now it really isn't an issue any more. Take the following smoothie for breakfast and/or dinner as often as possible and reduce your intake of alcohol, tomatoes, tobacco, peppers, aubergine (egg plant), orange juice and dairy produce. I genuinely hope you get a degree of relief from your condition.

2 **apples** (organic if possible – Royal Gala or Golden Delicious are nice)
1 handful **spinach**
¼ medium **cucumber**
1 stick **celery**
½ **avocado** (ripe)
4 **ice** cubes

With the juicer still off, place one whole apple in your whole fruit juicer. Pack in the spinach, add the cucumber, break up the celery stick and add, then finish by placing the other apple on top. Juice the lot. Add the avocado to your blender and then add the ice and juice. Blend.

Look what's in it! Vitamins A, B1, B2, B3, B5, B6, C and E, potassium, pectin, boron, ellagic acid, carotenes, calcium, silicon, iron, essential fats, natural sugars, amino acids, chlorophyll, folic acid, copper, phosphorus, zinc, magnesium and riboflavin.

How will it help clear my skin? One of the best minerals for skin conditions is zinc and this smoothie has a great deal of this much-needed mineral in the avocado. The smoothie is also rich in essential natural fats. These fats are of paramount importance for getting and maintaining clear skin. Maintaining a diet balance of 80 per cent alkaline and 20 per cent acid is also important for clear skin.

Juicy boost

To boost the natural fats and zinc dosage, add 1 heaped teaspoon of Juice Master's Clear Skin Booster before blending. This is also extremely alkaline.

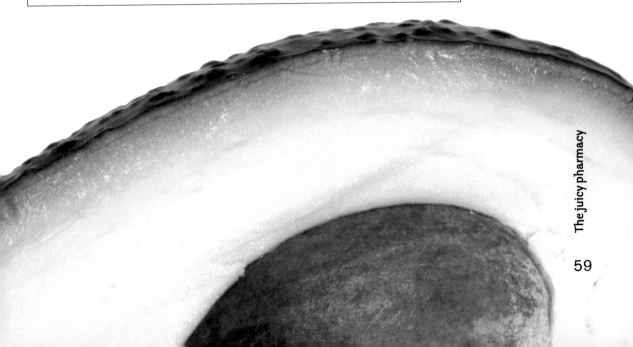

cellulite eliminator

Freshly extracted **apple, pear, celery** and **grapefruit** juice – all poured over **ice** and finished with some finely diced fresh **mint**

Beneath the skin is the subcutaneous layer, the purpose of which is to bind the skin to the bones or connective tissue beneath its surface. The subcutaneous layer is thinner in women than in men and as women age it becomes even thinner. It is because of this that fat cells become larger; they move closer to the skin's surface and show themselves in the bumpy form we have identified as cellulite. This doesn't mean nothing can be done. A poor diet and lack of exercise help to exacerbate this condition as it overloads the liver and lymphatic system with toxins. Get one of these smoothies inside you and a good dose of exercise and you should soon see a change.

1 **apple**
1 **pear**
¼ **pink grapefruit**
2 sticks of **celery**
A few **mint** leaves
4 **ice** cubes

Juice everything except the mint. Pour the juice into a glass over ice and sprinkle finely diced mint on top.

Look what's in it! Vitamins A, B, B1, B2, B6 and C, potassium, calcium, pectin, boron, ellagic acid, carotenes, amino acids, natural sugars, anti-oxidants, calcium, iron, sulphur, phosphorus, magnesium and malic acid.

How will it help me get rid of my cellulite? The apple and mint in this juice help to eliminate toxins from the fat tissue. The grapefruit has a high vitamin C content and is an excellent cleanser for a clogged lymphatic system. The celery, apple and pear juice help to cleanse the subcutaneous tissues and improve kidney function. All in all, this is much more effective than external creams – I believe in beauty care from within.

❛I recently bought a juicer and am now mad on it! I lost a stone in weight in just under 3 weeks! And that was not really why I started. I had headaches most evenings and hay fever allergies, etc., etc. ... anyway my headaches have gone and so has everything else. I feel great. ❜

Mary

ease the pressure

The **fresh** juice of sweet **cantaloupe** and **kiwi** fruit juice, mixed with **sodium-rich celery** juice, all **blended** together with **blackberries** and **ice**

Of all cases of high blood pressure 85 per cent are treatable without drugs! This comes as no surprise since the biggest cause of high blood pressure is poor diet and lifestyle. High blood pressure can lead to heart attacks and/or strokes, so sorting this problem out is extremely important. The good news is that with a change of diet and a few of these juices, all should be well.

Please Note: If you are already taking medication for high blood pressure, continue to do so and if you feel things are getting better ask your GP if you can come off them.

¼ cantaloupe **melon** (ripe)
4 **kiwi** fruit (gold or normal)
1 large handful **blackberries** (fresh or frozen)
1 stick **celery**
1 handful **ice**

You can juice a melon with the skin on (depending on your juicer), but sometimes the texture can be too thick if you do that. For this recipe I would advise scooping out the seeds and then scooping out the flesh before juicing. The same can be done with the kiwi fruit, although they can be juiced as they are. Juice the lot and pour over ice.

Look what's in it! Vitamins A, C and E, folic acid, potassium, iron, beta-carotene, calcium, magnesium, phosphorus, soluble fibre, anti-oxidants, natural sugars and amino acids.

How will it ease my blood pressure? This juice is loaded with vitamin C and calcium, both of which help to keep blood pressure at a normal level. It is thought that people who have a lot of potassium in their diets can help to reduce their medication dosage for high blood pressure. Celery is an excellent inner-body cleanser as well as being extremely calming for the nervous system; it also helps to rebuild red blood cells.

Juicy Note: If high blood pressure is not brought under control it can lead to heart attacks or strokes – so cut out the rubbish and get juicing ASAP!

breathe easy

Freshly extracted apple, carrot and lemon juice over ice

I suffered badly from asthma from the age of 8 until the age of 28. I was using the blue Ventolin inhaler up to 14 times a day and the brown steroid-based inhaler once a day. I am more than aware of the pain that asthma, or any type of breathing-related condition, can cause. I am not suggesting that the following recipe will 'cure' your asthma or whatever breathing problem you may have, but if you cut out all e-number foods and drinks, cut down on animal products (red meat and dairy mostly), step up your swimming and yoga (both very good for breathing conditions) and drink some freshly extracted juice every day, you will certainly breathe a lot easier.

2 **apples** (Golden Delicious or Royal Gala)
2 **carrots** (preferably organic – the darker orange the better)
1 inch slice **lemon** with rind on (unwaxed and organic if possible)
ice cubes

Juice the lot and pour over ice – that's it!

Look what's in it! Vitamin A, B, B1, B2, B6, C, E and K, beta-carotene, calcium, iron, magnesium, phosphorus, potassium, sulphur, amino acids, anti-oxidants, natural sugars, pectin and boron.

How will it help me to breathe more easily? Apples contain a compound called quercetin, which is a natural anti-histamine and is thought to help reduce the risk of asthma attacks. The remainder of the ingredients are packed with vitamin C, magnesium and vitamin E – all of which are beneficial for asthma sufferers. Researchers have found that people with a higher magnesium intake have healthier airways; it is also believed to protect against asthma by helping the muscles of the airways relax.

Juicy tip

Drop tea and coffee and replace with either hot water with lemon or peppermint tea. Getting rid of the milk will go a long way to helping you breathe, together with a dose of swimming every day.

arthritic relief

Creamy **pineapple**, grapefruit, **apple**, cucumber and **ginger** juice all blended together with fresh **blackberries** and **ice**

To a varying degree, over 80 per cent of people over the age of 50 show signs of this disorder, yet it is virtually unknown in the wild animal kingdom. Yes, dogs and cats get arthritic conditions, but they're not wild — we feed them! Wild animals consume only raw natural foods and this clearly plays a large role in keeping their joints in order. There have been many studies which show a clear link between certain foods and drinks and a flare up of osteoarthritis. My short piece of advice is to skip the solanum (nightshade) family — cooked tomatoes, aubergine, bell peppers, tobacco — as research has shown that certain substances found in these foods (and in tobacco) get in the way of normal collagen repair in the joints and/or promote inflammatory degeneration. Other foods to cut down on or skip altogether are dairy products, oranges, refined sugar (that's a big one), and excessive alcohol and red meat consumption. Do that and have this juice once a day and you'll be amazed at how the body, given the chance, can begin to heal.

Juicy boost

For a vitamin B12 boost, simply add 1 teaspoon of Juice Master's Ultimate Juice Boost before blending with the ice.

¼ **grapefruit** (pink or white)
¼ **pineapple** (fairtrade if you can)
1 **apple** (Royal Gala, Golden Delicious, or whatever you fancy – no Granny Smiths!)
1 small handful **blackberries**
1 inch slice **cucumber**
½ inch fresh **ginger**
ice cubes

Juice all the fruit and veg and pour over the ice. Drink slowly and enjoy!

Juicy Note: When juicing the blackberries, place the apple in first, then pack the blackberries in and turn on the machine. Feed the other ingredients in afterwards – you will get more juice that way.

Look what's in it! Vitamins A, B, B1, B2, B6 and C, calcium, iron, magnesium, phosphorus, folic acid, potassium, sulphur, amino acids, anti-oxidants, pectin, bromeline, malic acid, natural sugars and sodium.

How will this help ease my joints? Studies have shown that an intake of B vitamins and folic acid help to relieve stiffness in the joints of the hand. This recipe is loaded with a good supply of B vitamins and has folic acid from the blackberries. The bromeline in pineapples and the acids in grapefruits are of great benefit to certain arthritic conditions. Another great idea is simply to juice equal amounts of pineapple and grapefruit!

The juicy pharmacy

the unblocker

Fresh **apple, lemon** and **pear** juice all blended together with **pitted prunes** and **ice**

It's a subject in Britain we just don't like to talk about — constipation. We don't like to talk about it yet we are perhaps the most 'blocked' nation in Europe, with an extraordinary number of cases of bowel cancer a year. This is no surprise since our intake of lifeless and waterless foods plus the chemically packed drinks we ingest daily, soon leave their mark — and leave their mark is precisely what they do. Bits of sticky waterless food get stuck in our colon and can stay there for weeks, months and even years. There was one famous case where a woman who had been vegetarian for over 10 years had a colonic irrigation and traces of meat were discovered. That's 10 years after she stopped eating meat! The Unblocker is like super-strength Mr Muscle Sink Unblocker — but for the colon. If you can't 'go' then this powerful smoothie will have you reaching for the 'puppies on a roll' in no time.

2 **apples** (Golden Delicious or Royal Gala)
1 **pear** (Conference is best)
1 inch slice **lemon** with rind on (unwaxed if possible)
3 **prunes** (pitted and soaked overnight)
6 cubes **ice**

Juice the apples, pear and lemon. Pour into the blender with the pitted prunes and add ice. Blend until smooth and drink slowly. You may find that it takes a while to get the prunes smooth, depending on your blender, but it's OK if it's slightly 'bitty'.

Look what's in it! Vitamins B1, B2, B6 and C, pectin, beta-carotene, magnesium, phosphorus, sulphur, malic acid, iron, niacin, natural sugars, anti-oxidants and amino acids.

How will it clear the passage ahead? Prunes are the most famous natural laxative on Mother Earth. The apples and pear provide a tremendous amount of soluble fibre in the form of pectin which, when combined with the powerful laxative properties of prunes, help to unblock the most stubborn of situations (so to speak). Pear juice is well known in juicing circles for helping to protect the colon. The niacin (vitamin B3) and thiamine (vitamin B1) aid in the functioning of the nervous system and assist in proper blood formation and in the production of hydrochloric acid, which is important for proper digestion. They also help to lower 'bad' cholesterol levels. This smoothie is not for the faint hearted, as it has a sweet and sour taste about it. However, taste is not what this has been designed for — it's to 'take a weight off your mind'!

sexy juice

what we put into our body has an effect on how we move our body ... And that's every part!

We British don't really like to talk about Sex, and with more and more people losing their libido, it appears there's not much to talk about anyway! There are many contributing factors to lack of sex drive but without doubt what we put into our body has an effect on how we move our body ... And that's every part!

The following juicy recipes have been designed to put a little lead back in the ole pencil, a little libido back in your life. Let's put things into perspective here. If you are having significant problems in this area, please don't expect one shot of sexy juice to 'awaken the giant within' or get your juices flowing. If you want that sort of instant result you will need to say hello to Mr Viagra!

All of the following 'sexy juice' recipes contain ingredients that are said to have aphrodisiac and biological properties that can, as part of a balanced healthy lifestyle, improve performance in this area when consumed on a regular basis.

Please Note: The sexy juice recipes are good, but if you are drinking 10 pints of lager and expect a juice to help lift you out of trouble, I'm afraid you have more chance of flying to the moon on a cheese biscuit!

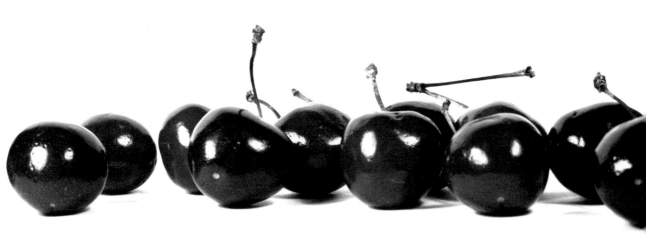

viagra relief

This recipe has been designed for all those who are looking to avoid ever having to take Viagra – which would be a relief to those concerned! This juice has several ingredients that help in this area.

¼ **pineapple**
1 large handful **raspberries**
100g low-fat live **yogurt**
4 **ice** cubes

Juice the pineapple and pour into the blender. Add the raspberries, yogurt and ice and blend.

Look what's in it! Zinc, zinc, zinc plus vitamins C and E, beta-carotene, potassium, iron, fibre, calcium, ellagic acid, natural sugars, amino acids and anti-oxidants.

How will it juice me? Zinc is the nutrient most associated with sex, for three principal reasons. It is the nutrient which governs testosterone, which is needed for sperm production. A woman's body prepares herself for sex more quickly if zinc levels are high and human sperm is packed with it – if a man were to have sex just three times in 24 hours his entire zinc supply would be depleted. A high content of zinc is found in the seeds of raspberries and as, unlike most fruits, these seeds are eaten in full, you benefit from the full amount of zinc.

strawberry heaven

A rather crude name, I appreciate, but it is justified. The high zinc content of fresh strawberries means someone is in for a treat, in more ways than one!

¼ medium **pineapple**
1 large handful fresh **strawberries**
100g low-fat live **yogurt**
4 **ice** cubes

Juice the pineapple and pour into the blender. Add the strawberries, yogurt and ice. Blend the lot until smooth.

Look what's in it! Vitamins C and E, ellagic acid, folic acid, beta-carotene, potassium, iron, zinc, pro-biotics, calcium, amino acids, natural sugars and anti-oxidants.

How will it juice me? Strawberries are the king of zinc in the fruit world and zinc is the one mineral that does more for your libido than any other. The high vitamin C content is excellent for cleaning the liver and kidneys.

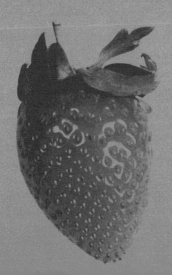

Sexyjuice

73

berry va va voom

Blueberries and live yogurt blended with delicious extracted orange juice and ice

Blueberries are a berry known for giving an extra nutritional injection into your love life. This smoothie not only tastes sweet and creamy, but has been designed to add a little 'Va Va Voom' in the bedroom (or wherever else takes your fancy!)

1 handful fresh **blueberries**
1 large **orange** (peeled but with the pith on)
100g low-fat live **yogurt**
4 **ice** cubes

Juice the orange and pour into the blender. Add the blueberries, yogurt and ice. Blend until creamy and smooth.

Look what's in it! Vitamins B1, B2, B6 and C, calcium, magnesium, phosphorus, sodium, beta-carotene, ellagic acid, folic acid, iron, potassium, zinc, friendly bacteria, amino acids, anti-oxidants and natural sugars.

How will it juice me? Blueberries are once again high in the performance-enhancing mineral, zinc. This smoothie also contains ellagic acid, an anti-ageing phytochemical, so not only will you perform better in the bedroom but you could live longer — so enjoy more of it.

Juicy factoid

It is said that if a man eats a handful of blueberries before he has sex, his sperm will taste a whole lot sweeter!

‘ Since starting the juicing program, I've lost weight, I look great, I feel great, and I'm bursting with energy for the first time in 15 years. I've never been happier. For the paltry price of a juicer and your book, my life has changed completely. ’

Tony

love tonic

This is a dairy-free Love Tonic. All the other recipes in this section have included yogurt, so for all you vegans out there, here's a love tonic that meets your needs without an animal product in sight.

½ fresh medium **pineapple**
1 handful **raspberries**
1 handful **strawberries**
4 **ice** cubes

Juice the pineapple and pour into the blender. Add the raspberries, strawberries and ice. Blend until creamy and smooth.

Look what's in it Vitamins C and E, calcium, iron, sodium, zinc, potassium, phosphorus, beta-carotene, ellagic acid, fibre, natural sugars, amino acids, sulphur, niacin and folic acid.

How will it juice me? Zinc once again is the key mineral here for helping to boost libido. The two berries contain large amounts of this lovemaking enhancing super-mineral.

the quickie

Sometimes you're just in the mood for a quickie, so with that in mind this is one for such occasions. No juicer needed for this recipe; just blend the ingredients and BOOM! You're done. This is quick to make, quick to take effect and is the perfect libido lift if you want a quickie…so to speak.

1 handful **strawberries**
½ **banana**
100g low-fat live **yogurt**
1 tablespoon **tahini**
ice cubes

Simply put all ingredients into the blender and blend until smooth.

Look what's in it! Rich in zinc, B vitamins, folic acid, vitamins A, C and E, potassium, friendly bacteria, calcium, linoleic acids, sodium, magnesium and fibre.

How will it juice me? The high potassium content of this smoothie is ideal for any kind of physical activity. This smoothie is full of sex-drive-enhancing zinc, so it is perfect for topping up your zinc level.

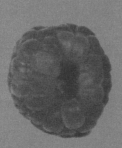

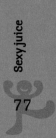

natural beauty

'If we eat rubbish, chances are we will look like rubbish too!'

In the UK hundreds of millions of pounds is spent on all sorts of ways to try and make ourselves look beautiful on the outside. Anything from simple make-up to voluntarily paralysing our faces with botox! It appears that no matter how insane it is, we will try just about anything to get the body and face beautiful. When I say 'anything', I mean anything apart from actually changing what we eat and drink on a regular basis.

Adding the latest external 'age-defying' lotion to your body in an attempt to look amazing is like putting paint on rust to make it look nice. The bottom line is that 'beauty comes from within', and the biggest change externally happens when you change things internally.

Nature provides all the elements needed keep your body and face beautiful in the 'living' food she grows for us. Even the finest external applications are to be found amongst nature's finest. Cucumbers for tired eyes and ripe avocado for use as a face pack to tighten and supply moisture back into the skin. However, the real beauty comes when we start to pour some of this super food into our systems.

So, whether you're looking for hard nails, radiant skin, bright eyes, shiny hair or just a bit of a glow, the following juicy recipes should help do the trick.

> 'Just had to share my delight with you … I have lost 18lbs in 14 days! My husband looks and feels 10 years younger and is even spreading the word to his 'food police' mates. I overheard him explaining to one that 'juicing isn't a diet, it's a permanent change of lifestyle'.'
>
> Alison

hard as nails

Fresh blueberries and blackberries blended together with almonds, banana and ice and finished with finely diced mint

As the title suggests, the ingredients in this quick and simple, natural beauty smoothie are all there to help strengthen your nails. Did you know that your finger nails grow four times as fast as your toe nails? Well, you do now. As with all the recipes produced from nature's liquid fuel, they will help the overall health and strength of the body, not just specific parts. You might also be pleased to know that you don't even need your juicer for this natural beauty smoothie, just your blender (so much easier to clean!).

1 small handful **almonds** (soaked overnight)
1 small handful **blueberries**
1 small handful **blackberries**
4 **ice** cubes
1 small **banana**
1 pinch fresh **mint**
¼ cup **mineral water**

Simply put everything, except the mint, into the blender and blend for 45 seconds or until smooth. Dice the mint and add to the smoothie once poured.

Please Note: Unless you have a Vitamix blender (very expensive!) the chances are you won't fully blend the almonds. This just means the smoothie will be crunchier – delicious!

Look what's in it! Vitamins A, B1, B2, B3, B6, C and E, calcium, phosphorus, potassium, magnesium, iron, sodium, zinc, folic acid, amino acids, natural sugars and 'good' essential fats.

How will it juice my nails? Almonds are one of the only alkalizing nuts around and as such help to level the body's alkaline/acid balance. They also contain essential oils and trace minerals, such as magnesium, which are excellent for the strengthening, growth and repair of the nails. Blueberries and blackberries are packed with B vitamins and folic acid. They are well known for helping the body to work as a whole and maintain a natural balance – and they also taste wonderful! Bananas are one of the richest sources of potassium in the world and are an excellent source of amino acids (the building blocks for protein). The combination of their vitamins, minerals and amino acids make bananas an excellent nail and bone builder. Mint is a good decongestant, but it's been added here just to add a little extra taste.

skin deep

Freshly extracted apple, cucumber and celery juice blended with avocado, brazil nuts and ice

Having suffered from psoriasis and eczema myself, I am well aware that one juice will not cut the mustard for conditions such as that. However, having researched this subject for well over a decade, I have come up with this excellent combination that will go a long way towards improving skin tone, elasticity and many skin conditions.

½ **avocado**
6 **Brazil** nuts
¼ **cucumber**
¼ stick **celery**
4 large **apples** (Royal Gala for preference)
ice cubes

Cut an avocado in half, remove the stone, scoop out flesh from one half and put into blender, along with ice and Brazil nuts. Juice the rest, add to blender and blend for 45 seconds or until smooth.

Juicy boost

To help this juice reach the parts of you that other juices can't, simply add a teaspoon of Juice Master's Clear Skin Booster before blending.

Look what's in it! Vitamins A, B, B1, B2, B3, B5, B6, C and E, riboflavin, iron, calcium, copper, phosphorus, zinc, magnesium, folic acid, beta-carotene, selenium, lecithin and essential fatty acids.

How will it juice my skin? Brazil nuts contain lecithin, selenium and essential fatty acids, all of which are essential for good elasticity of the skin and a glowing complexion. The lecithin in the Brazil nuts is a natural fat emulsifier and as such helps the body to absorb the essential fats it needs for good skin. Cucumbers are excellent for rejuvenating muscles and are also superb for giving back elasticity to the skin. In addition, they are perhaps the best natural diuretic known to wo/mankind and are simply excellent for any skin problem. Celery juice helps to flush the system of excessive carbon dioxide, which plays a part in the body's largest organ – the skin. Apple juice is not just refreshing, but is excellent for cleaning the colon and promoting good-looking skin. Avocado contains essential fatty acids (in omega oil form), which all help to promote excellent skin.

Juicy tip

Brazil nuts might not blend smooth (depending on your blender), so soak them first and don't be put off if this smoothie has an extra crunch to it.

---

bright eyes

The eyes tell a great deal about someone's health and when you see big bright eyes it's usually a good sign that things are working well internally. However, as well as having bright eyes, it also helps to be able to see out of them too! With that in mind, the following recipe has been designed to not only brighten your eyes but also to add a little 20/20 to your day.

½ medium **pineapple**
2 **carrots**
1 handful fresh flat-leaved **parsley**
1 small handful fresh **mint**
ice cubes

Juice the pineapple, carrots and parsley. Dice a small amount of fresh mint and add to the juice. Add ice to cool.

Look what's in it! Vitamins A, B, C, D, E and K, iron, folic acid, potassium, calcium, magnesium, manganese and natural sugars.

How will it juice my eyes? Carrot juice has incredible power in improving night vision and eyesight in general. Parsley juice, when combined with carrot, has even greater healing properties than carrot alone. This powerful herb can be used for weak eyes, cataracts, conjunctivitis and laziness of the pupil. Dull eyes are usually the first sign that things aren't right within and pineapple juice has the amazing ability to clear mucus whilst supplying the body with live nutrients, all helping your eyes to shine white and bright. Mint contains oils, flavonoids and menthol, once again helping to flush the system and so promote bright eyes. Mint also makes it taste good.

one for the hair

They say that if you don't wash your hair for a time your hair will start to clean itself with its own natural oils. I have only one piece of advice on that one – **don't do it!** I tried it and just ended up with hair that looked like it hadn't been properly washed for weeks (which is precisely what it was!). The only advice I would give is to have one of the following and wash your hair.

½ small **cucumber**
1 cup **alfalfa sprouts**
2 **brussels sprouts**
2 large **carrots**
2 large **apples** (Royal Gala for preference)
1 inch fresh **ginger**
ice cubes

Simply juice the lot and add some ice to cool.

Look what's in it! Vitamins A, B1, B2, B3, B5 , B6, C, D, E and K, iron, potassium, magnesium, calcium, folic acid, beta-carotene, sulphur, silicon, phyto-oestrogens and natural sugars.

How will it juice my hair? Alfalfa sprouts are rich in phyto-oestrogens, which help to counteract the excessive stimulating effect of male hormones on the hair follicles. They are rich in silicon, excellent for the growth of strong and healthy hair. Brussels sprouts and ginger are high in organic sulphur, which stimulates the growth of healthy hair. Carrots contain beta-carotene, essential to reduce inflammation in the scalp. Cucumber is a magnificent cleanser and body cooler. It is a rich source of many trace minerals essential for maintaining a healthy head of hair.

juice master's ultimate health booster

Don't let ingredients like 'broccoli' or 'watercress' put you off here. I try to create juices which are both excellent for health and your tastebuds! This 'beauty juice' not only tastes sweet and creamy, due to a high percentage of apple and pineapple juice combined with avocado, but it contains just about everything your body and mind require for outstanding beauty. All of the ingredients help to cleanse the system, feed the cells and boost the immune system. As beauty and health come from within, this liquid sunshine will have you looking good, feeling good in no time at all.

1 inch slice **pineapple**

1 **apple** (Royal Gala or Golden Delicious are best)

1 inch chunk **broccoli** stem

1 small handful **spinach**

½ stick **celery**

¼ inch piece **ginger** (with skin on)

1 inch slice **cucumber**

1 small handful **watercress**

Parsley (just a small amount – it's quite a powerful herb. Leave out if you have kidney problems or are pregnant)

½ ripe **avocado** (de-stoned)

ice cubes

Juice everything except the avocado. Place the avocado in the blender along with the ice and add juice. Blend until smooth – enjoy!

Look what's in it! Vitamins A, B, B2, B3, B5, B6 and C, folic acid, chlorophyll, sulphur, magnesium, calcium, iron, silicon, potassium, beta-carotene, boron, ellagic acid, phosphorus, chlorine, iodine, sodium, natural sugars, natural fats, zinc and copper.

How will it juice me? Pineapple juice has anti-inflammatory properties, supports the digestion of proteins and acts as a mild laxative and diuretic. It also reduces mucus congestion, making it excellent for bronchitis and asthma. Apple juice helps to soothe the intestines and, like pineapple, reduces constipation. It helps to wipe out unfriendly bacteria and parasites within the digestive tract. Broccoli is one of the most powerful anti-oxidants in the world. It contains vitamins B and C, folic acid, beta-carotene, phosphorus, calcium, potassium and iodine. It is superb for blood pressure and liver problems. Spinach juice is a must ingredient – it heals the lining of the digestive tract, improves vision and reduces arthritic pain. It also helps to maintain healthy blood vessels and is packed with the 'liquid sunshine' of the veggie world – chlorophyll. Celery juice is a natural diuretic, which reduces fluid retention. It is also the best natural source of sodium on the planet. Ginger is a natural antibiotic which adds a little kick to this incredible juice. Cucumber juice is the super-cooler of the natural world and is excellent for cooling the body, flushing excess wastes and improving the skin. Watercress is a mineral marvel – sulphur, calcium, iron, sodium, magnesium, phosphorus, chlorine, potassium and iodine are all in this one juice. Parsley is incredibly high in iron and chlorophyll and helps to maintain healthy blood vessels and eyes. It is an excellent cleanser of the liver, kidneys and blood.

juicy h₂o

Light, refreshing, scrummy and good for you — water never tasted so great!

Sometimes a juice or smoothie can be a little too much for your needs and water is sometimes, well, boring! With that in mind I have created this refreshing thirst-quenching array of natural Juicy Waters.

There are now many juicy waters in the shops, but beware — they nearly all have sugar or artificial sweeteners in! As always, you can't top making your own. Fresh is the winner every time. The ONLY one in the shops I would recommend at this time is the juicy water range from our friends at Innocent, but even these have some sugar added.

This small selection of juicy waters are also excellent for diabetics as undiluted juices aren't really recommended, unless they are of the veggie kind. When a smoothie is too thick and a juice is too filling, Juice Master's Juicy H_2Os will quench even the most insatiable thirsts. ENJOY!

water, water everywhere, but …

Clearly, all of the juicy water recipes in this section use water as the main base. However, not all water is the same and there are many waters on the market today. The bottom line is we are in the fortunate position of being in a developed country. This means that, although many people in this country treat tap water like it's the

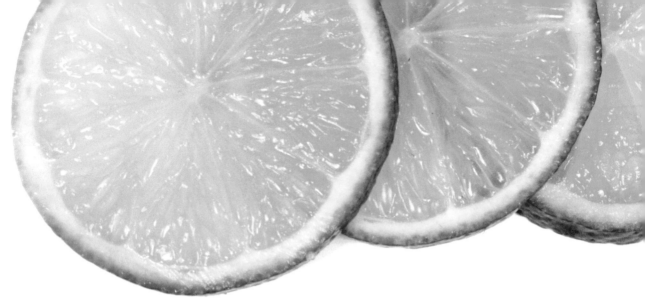

most contaminated substance on earth, in fact it is perfectly clean and perfectly fine. While there are some nasties in it, on the whole it will do a great deal more good than harm – just try not having any water for a while! Having said that, I still choose to drink mineral water most of the time since I can afford it and it doesn't contain the few nasties that tap water does.

Bizarrely, spring water is not in fact a mineral water and some waters labelled 'spring' can come directly from the tap. Mineral water is water which has been naturally filtered through rock formations and then bottled at source. It is the most common of all water sold in this country and the one I personally use. Although this type of water contains minerals they are inorganic, and this means that those not utilized – most of them – will simply be flushed out of the body. So you will be having this water for the mountain water and not for the minerals. Reverse Osmosis (RO) works by filtering water through a semi-permeable membrane that won't allow most contaminates to pass through. The system isn't perfect, as typically it will only filter 5–15 per cent of the water entering the system, but I would always choose it over spring water.

flavoured waters

Nearly all 'flavoured waters' will have either artificial flavours or colours and I would steer clear of them all. The same goes for 'sports waters', which tend to contain artificial sweetners and/or sugar. If in doubt, check the label carefully.

h₂o refresher

Sometimes you want something cool, refreshing and good for you. When you read what the H$_2$O Refresher has in it and what it can do, you will see just how amazing it is. Just as refreshing as water, but with all the live goodness of nature.

½ litre mineral **water** (or your choice of water)
1 inch thick slice **watermelon** (straight from the fridge)

Simply juice the watermelon and dilute with water to taste.

Look what's in it! Folic acid, potassium, vitamins A, C and E, iron, beta-carotene, calcium, magnesium and phosphorus – and those are the nutrients and minerals found in the watermelon. You may be using mineral water, but remember, you can't really count those minerals as they are mainly inorganic and the body simply cannot utilize them.

How will it juice me? Watermelon is one of the most cooling and refreshing fruits in the world. It is one of only a fairly small number of fruits which contain vitamin E. This vitamin is important in the prevention of cardiovascular disease, it helps reduce blood pressure and it even helps to prevent anaemia. The vitamin A will help to maintain healthy skin, eyes and bones. Watermelon has been used in the treatment of many diseases, including the prevention of certain cancers.

Juicy Note: As cleaning the juicer can be seen by some as a right royal pain in the proverbial, it is worth making any other juice you are going to have at the same time. So if you want this juicy H$_2$O for a day after lying in the sun (great coolant) or just a refreshing drink, make another one at the same time and keep it in your juicy flask.

h₂o cool

About as cooling as it gets! The expression, 'cool as a cucumber' came about for a reason. In some of the hottest countries on Earth you will find this wonderful veggie-fruit bathing in the blazing midday sun. Despite this they remain cool to the touch and are up there with watermelon and celery in their ability to cool the inner body. With that in mind it comes as no surprise that cucumber is one of the main ingredients in the H_2O Cool.

½ litre mineral **water** (or your choice of water)
¼ **cucumber**
½ **apple** (Golden Delicious or Royal Gala are best)

Juice the cucumber and apple and simply dilute with water. If you wish to keep the juice for a while, just to squeeze a bit of lemon into it.

Look what's in it! Vitamins A, B, B1, B2, B3, B5, B6 and C, folic acid, calcium, chlorine, iron, potassium, silicon, boron, ellagic acid, carotenes and natural sugars.

How will it juice me? Instant body cooler and thirst quencher, this Juicy H_2O is great for rejuvenating muscles, giving elasticity to the skin and helps to promote hair and fingernail growth and prevent hair loss. It is also an excellent diuretic, powerful anti-oxidant, improving brain and nerve function and stimulating the immune system – not bad for a juicy water!

h$_2$o lift

This Juicy H$_2$O has been designed to lift the body, mind and soul. Don't be fooled by the seemingly sparse ingredients in this juicy water; as with any of nature's finest, even a diluted tiny amount can have a powerful effect.

½ litre mineral **water** (or your choice of water)
1 juicy **orange** (peeled but keep pith on – that's where the goodness is)
1 inch thick slice medium **pineapple**
1 squeeze **lime**

Juice the orange and pineapple, dilute with water and squeeze in the lime.

Look what's in it! Vitamins B1, B6 and C, calcium, folic acid, iron, potassium and bioflavonoids.

How will it juice me? Vitamin B1, otherwise known as thiamine, is involved in the release of energy from carbohydrates – just perfect for H$_2$O Lift. Vitamin B6 (pyridoxine) is involved in more bodily functions than almost any other single nutrient. It's great for water retention, helps red blood cell formation and is important for maintaining a healthy nervous system. This juicy H$_2$O also contains calcium, which is excellent for reducing acid in the body and, of course, great for the bones and teeth. Who would have thought that when you look at the ingredients!

zesty h$_2$o

Water with an edge! This is an extremely vibrant and refreshing water. The lemon and lime give it a real edge and it's certainly not for the faint-hearted. As with all the Juicy H$_2$Os, Zesty H$_2$O will not only hydrate but also nourish from top to toe. One of the main reasons you will love this recipe is **you don't have to use your juicer**! Yep, it's a case of squeeze and go …

½ litre mineral **water** (or your choice of water)
½ **lemon**
1 **lime**

Simply squeeze the lemon and lime and dilute with water.

Look what's in it! Vitamin C, beta-carotene, calcium, magnesium, bioflavonoids, potassium, anti-oxidants and folic acid.

How will it juice me? This apparently simple-looking juicy H$_2$O packs a healthy punch. The vitamin C helps increase activity of white blood cells, keeps tissues strong and healthy and sweeps up damaging free radicals. It will help to lower cholesterol, control blood pressure and aid the body's absorption of iron and calcium. As with all the Juicy H$_2$Os it contains natural sugars and live diluted nutrition.

h$_2$o red body tonic

All of the Juicy H$_2$Os can be described as nature's tonics, but this one in particular has been created to add a little more oomph than the others. One of the main ingredients is raw beetroot (trust me, it will taste divine!). Raw beetroot is one of the best natural blood builders on the planet and although it is about as tasty as an unbuttered cream cracker if drunk on its own, once diluted with some apple, lemon and a tiny amount of cucumber, it's as scrummy as all the rest.

½ litre mineral **water** (or your choice of water)
1 small **red beetroot** (must be RAW!)
¼ inch slice **cucumber**
1 **apple** (Golden Delicious or Royal Gala are best)
1 squeeze **lemon**
1 sports **bottle** or **flask**

Juice the beetroot, cucumber and apple, dilute with water and add the lemon. That's it!

Look what's in it! Vitamins A, B, B1, B2, B3, B5, B6 and C, folic acid, calcium, chlorine, manganese, iron, potassium, phosphorus, silicon, boron, ellagic acid, carotenoids and natural sugars.

How will it juice me? Great for the blood, this juice helps brain function and is good for the bones and sugar metabolism. Hydrating and an excellent natural diuretic, it will cleanse the kidneys. H_2O Red Body Tonic is a good laxative, easing constipation. It can even help to prevent the harshest of ailments such as cancer and heart disease (as long as you skip the cigs and doughnuts, of course!). Good for the nails, hair and skin, and a superb tonic if at all anaemic. This Juicy Water is very antibacterial and will help to fight infections.

Juicy tip

If you wish to keep the juice for a while, remember to squeeze a bit of lemon in it.

‘ Beetroot juice is one of the most valuable juices for helping to build up the red corpuscles of the blood and tone up the blood generally. ’

Dr Norman Walker (Juicing pioneer)

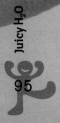

no sweat

fear not, my gym bunny friends, as anti-oxidants are found in every juice and smoothie in this book!

Exercise (love it or hate it) – if you want to look good, feel good and keep your bones and body healthy, you gotta do a bit here and there. However, even with something as beneficial as exercise, unless you get the right fuel, it can sometimes do more harm than good.

When you exercise you lose vital minerals and fluids and these need replacing as soon as possible. Excessive exercise also creates free radicals – atoms or groups of atoms containing at least one unpaired electron, which, wanting to be paired, steal electrons from other pairs. In layman's terms, if these unpaired electrons are free to roam they create a harmful imbalance in the body. So harmful in fact that these free radicals have been implicated in the development of diseases such as cancer and heart disease.

But fear not, my gym bunny friends, as anti-oxidants, found in every juice and smoothie in this book, attach themselves to these damaging molecules and neutralize the little suckers. All of the following recipes have been designed not only to mop up any free radical damage which may occur during exercise, but also to boost performance and recovery naturally.

The body requires optimum fuel for exercise and recovery. The following juicy recipes will meet all of your exercise and/or body-building needs — and not an isotonic drink in sight!

vegan protein power smoothie

freshly extracted **pineapple** and **apple** juice blended with **avocado, banana, spirulina** and **ice**

Whoever said you need animal products to build muscle? Oh yes, the people who are responsible for selling them! The biggest and most powerful land animals in the world are vegan (buffalo, elephant, giraffe, hippos, etc.), so clearly you don't need animal products for power and strength. The Vegan Protein Power Smoothie contains ALL of the essential amino acids (the building blocks for protein) required to build muscle. Not only that, as with all the recipes in the book it tastes pretty damn good too.

¼ small **pineapple**
2 **apples** (Golden Delicious or Royal Gala for preference)
½ ripe **avocado** (de-stoned and peeled)
1 medium **banana** (peeled)
¼ teaspoon **spirulina** (if you haven't got any just make without)
A few **ice** cubes

Cut up the pineapple so it fits in the feeder of your juicer and juice it along with the apples. Place the avocado in the blender along with the banana, spirulina, ice and the freshly extracted juice. Blend until smooth.

Look what's in it! Essential fats, ALL of the essential amino acids, natural sugars, fibre, vitamins A, B, B6, C and E, riboflavin, iron, calcium, copper, phosphorus, zinc, boron, niacin, magnesium, folic acid and carotenes. Not bad for a little smoothie with no animal products!

How will it juice me? Contains 10 times more calcium than milk and 58 times more iron than spinach! The essential amino acids contained within this vegan smoothie will help any budding body-builders out there. The zinc helps to protect the liver from chemical damage, is vital for bone formation and promotes a healthy immune system and the healing of wounds. Boron is needed for healthy bones and muscle growth because it assists in the production of natural steroid compounds within the body.

Juicy tip

Have a small glass about half an hour before exercise and again after exercise.

natural
performance enhancer

Creamy **banana**, **tahini** paste, live low-fat **yogurt** and **honey** blended with freshly extracted **pineapple** and **apple** juice and **ice**

In the world of sport, finding ways to enhance performance has led some athletes to, well, cheat. When I say cheat, I mean, of course, take performance-enhancing illegal drugs. I've added the word illegal because substances such as caffeine and refined sugars are stimulants too, yet the same rules don't apply. It appears to be perfectly OK to down a few Red Bulls before a competition, but take an illegal drug to help 'give you wings' and you are banned for life. Anyway, whether legal or not, natural is always best when it comes to performance enhancing and this excellent smoothie has been designed to do exactly what it says on the tin (so to speak) – enhance performance naturally.

¼ small **pineapple** (fairtrade if you can – every little helps)
1 **apple** (Golden Delicious or Royal Gala for preference)
½ **banana** (again, fairtrade if possible)
2 tablespoons **tahini paste** (pulped sesame seeds – can be purchased just about anywhere)
2 tablespoons live low-fat **yogurt**
1 teaspoon **Manuka active honey**
A few **ice** cubes

Cut the pineapple so it fits in the feeder of your juicer and juice it along with the apple. Place the banana, tahini paste, yogurt, Manuka honey, and ice into blender along with the apple and pineapple juice. Blend until smooth.

Look what's in it! Vitamins A, B1, B2, B6 and C, beta-carotene, potassium, fibre, folic acid, magnesium, boron, ellagic acid, calcium, iron, friendly bacteria, UMF® (Unique Manuka Factor), plus, of course, all the other magnificent elements nature has provided which we are yet to discover and name.

How will it juice me? The many natural sugars will provide an excellent source of carbohydrate fuel for the body. The natural live yogurt will act as a 'buffer' to prevent those sugars from being released into the bloodstream too quickly. This allows for a steady fuel release after an initial 'juice boost'. The 'unique Manuka factor' is related to the 'active' antibacterial properties of the Manuka honey, which is claimed to be the most powerful antibacterial food on Earth. Live nutrients, live yogurt and 'active' honey … the perfect ingredients to enhance performance naturally.

juice master's sports hydro juice

The only way to obtain a live sports drink with no artificial anything is to make it fresh yourself. Freshly extracted juices are hydrating, but sometimes smoothies and juices can be too 'heavy' for sporting needs. This specially formulated juice not only meets your water needs, but it also supplies your system with vital natural sugars and minerals which are lost during exercise.

¼ **cucumber**
¼ stick **celery**
1 small whole **beetroot**
½ **apple** (Golden Delicious or Royal Gala are best)
1 slice **lemon** (with rind on – if unwaxed)
½ litre mineral **water**

Simply juice the cucumber, celery, beetroot and apple and pour into a sports water bottle or a flask. Add the mineral water and lemon, shake and you're done!

Look what's in it! Vitamins B1, B2, B3, B5, B6 and C, folic acid, calcium, sodium, chlorine, iron, potassium, magnesium, bioflavonoids and beta-carotene.

How will it juice me? The perfect balance of sodium and potassium helps to prevent aches, pains, muscle cramps and lactic acid build-up. Potassium helps with proper muscle contraction and works with sodium to control the body's water balance. The cucumber helps to cool the system, the celery replaces lost sodium, the apple is known to help lower cholesterol and the lemon adds some zest to the recipe whilst helping to cleanse the liver and kidneys.

Juicy Note: Unlike the 'Workout Wonder' – which has similar ingredients – the Sports Hydro Juice has been designed to be drunk before, during and after exercise. It will taste more like water than juice, but it will enable you to perform 33 per cent longer than water alone and your recovery will be much faster too. This recipe is perfect for during a marathon or triathlon.

workout wonder

This juice combination is said, by juice pioneers old and new, to be the perfect balance of sodium and potassium – ideal for pre and post-exercise. It is one of the most popular juices in Juice Master Juice 'n' Smoothie bars up and down the country, and is the 'thick' version, if you will, of the Juice Master's Sports Hydro Juice. It is also one of the easiest juices to make.

¼ **cucumber**

1 stick **celery**

2 **apples** (Golden Delicious or Royal Gala are best)

¼ **lemon** (rind on – if waxed just peel first. This isn't in our juice bar version but it is ideal for helping to prevent the juice oxidizing if taking to the gym in a juicy flask)

Simply juice the cucumber, celery, apples and lemon and pour over ice. If taking to the gym, fill to top of flask and close.

Look what's in it! Vitamins B1, B2, B3, B5, B6 and C, iron, potassium, sodium, chlorine, magnesium, bioflavonoids, beta-carotene, folic acid and calcium.

How will it juice me? The perfect balance of sodium and potassium helps to prevent the build up of lactic acid and cramps, as well as replacing natural salts. The celery in the juice also helps to flush the body of excessive carbon dioxide. As well as being superb for athletes this juice is helpful for arthritis sufferers as it helps reduce acidity in the body.

Juicy Note: I often make twice the amount of this juice, drink a small glass while on my way to the gym and put the rest in my juicy flask. I then drink the rest slowly in a gorgeous sauna! If you are a member of Virgin Active you may well see a Juice Master Juice Bar there; if so you can save yourself the trouble of making it yourself and have it as fresh as it gets!

No sweat

rapid recovery

Blueberries, banana and ice blended with delicious freshly extracted pineapple, celery, cucumber, apple and lime juice

Whether you are building up your sweat by running, cycling, aerobics, weight-lifting, body-pumping or whatever, the Rapid Recovery will make sure you don't spend the next 3 days not being able to move! Full of natural sugars, sodium, vitamins, minerals, essential fats, amino acids and anti-oxidants, the Rapid Recovery has everything to help your depleted and tired bod return to normal in super-fast time.

¼ medium **pineapple**
½ stick **celery**
1 inch thick slice **cucumber**
1 **apple** (Golden Delicious or Royal Gala are best)
1 **lime** (peeled)
¼ cup **blueberries**
½ **banana**
4 **ice** cubes

Cut the pineapple so it fits into chute of juicer. (You can leave the skin on or take it off – your choice. Not all juice extractors will juice pineapple well with the skin still on. If you have the Philips wide-chute juicer then you can leave it on). Juice the celery, cucumber, apple, lime and pineapple and pour into the blender along with the ice, blueberries and banana. Blend until smooth, pour and drink slowly.

Look what's in it! Vitamins A, B, B1, B2, B6, C and E, potassium, sodium, boron, calcium, zinc, ellagic acid, folic acid, beta-carotene, silicon, phosphorus, tannins, magnesium, iron, bioflavonoids, natural sugars, natural fats, fibre and, of course, plenty of anti-oxidants.

How will it juice me? The tremendous amount of anti-oxidants will help to mop up any 'free radicals' which may be causing problems due to strenuous exercise. In fact, ellagic acid, which is found in blueberries, is one of the most powerful weapons against free radical damage. The high potassium content in the Rapid Recovery is important for a healthy nervous system and helps to keep the heart rhythm regular, as well as maintaining stable blood pressure. Blueberries, although more understated than the now 'hip and trendy' acai berry, is just as, if not even more, beneficial to overall health, and is one of nature's top body healers.

Juicy Note: Although all of the juices and smoothies in this 'No Sweat' section are more than capable of helping the body when it comes to exercise and recovery, Rapid Recovery has been carefully designed to do what it says, feed the body everything it requires to repair, heal and build after a sweaty session.

simple, gorgeous smoothies

pure liquid engineering for your body and mind...

Unlike juices, smoothies contain the fibres of the fruits as well as the juice. This is why you should never have a smoothie with a meal as it is a meal in itself. Personally I LOVE smoothies. The texture, the taste, the fact they are incredibly filling and yet so unbelievably good for you. However, not all smothies are all they appear to be on the health front, so when out and about — watch out!

When you buy smoothies in juice bars, most of the time you are getting a combination of pasteurized juice and some sugar-loaded yogurt with a bit of fresh or frozen fruit thrown in to give the impression that all is well and healthy. A recent article in *The Times* pointed out that one particular smoothie from a famous juice bar chain was over 1400 calories — yes just one smoothie! The man who wrote the article made the comment that 'at least Burger King is honest' — when people go into a juice bar they believe they are getting something healthy, whereas Burger King don't even try to pretend.

The only way to guarantee a gorgeous and amazingly healthy smoothie is either to find a decent, genuine juice bar (see www.juicemaster.com for a list) or, better still, to make it yourself – at least that way you know exactly what is going into it.

The following recipes have been carefully designed not only to satisfy your taste buds, but also your appetite and your health bank account – enjoy!

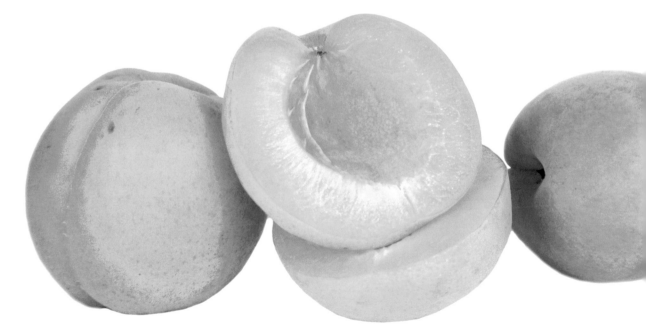

simply divine

Thick, freshly extracted mango and orange juice blended together with fresh strawberries and crushed ice

Picture lying down on a white sandy beach, the sun beating down, and sipping an ice-cold creamy fruit cocktail. If you close your eyes when drinking this divine smoothie, it is possible to forget where you are and transport yourself for a few minutes.

1 **mango** (de-stoned)
1 **orange** (peeled but with pith on)
1 small handful **strawberries**
1 small handful crushed **ice**

Juice the mango and orange. Put the strawberries and ice in the blender along with the juice. Blend – pour – enjoy!

Smoothie benefits Rich in vitamins B, C and E, and loaded with zinc, iron, calcium and potassium. The zinc helps to maintain the proper concentration of vitamin E in the blood. The natural sugars give an energy lift.

a bit of a honey!

This smoothie really is a bit of a honey!

The sweet and creamy elixir of freshly extracted peach and pineapple juice combined with the understated flavour of fresh banana and accompanied by the delicious sweet nectar of Manuka 'active' honey.

- 1 **peach** (de-stoned)
- ¼ medium **pineapple**
- ⅓ **banana**
- 1 teaspoon **Manuka active honey** (if you can't get Manuka honey, substitute another sort)
- 1 small handful crushed **ice**

Juice only one half of the peach along with the pineapple. Pour into the blender along with the honey, banana, crushed ice and other half of the peach. Blend – pour – enjoy!

Smoothie benefits Bananas contain three natural sugars – sucrose, fructose and glucose – and combined with its fibre a banana gives an instant, sustained and substantial boost of energy. This smoothie is also very rich in potassium, iron and, thanks to the peach, vitamins A, B3 and C. The active ingredients in the Manuka honey add some serious antibacterial properties to this already powerful smoothie. Designed to keep you slim, trim and healthy – or a bit of a hunny, as they say!

tropical paradise

Fresh **pineapple** juice, puréed **banana** and luscious **mango**, blended with cool **coconut** milk

Quite simply paradise in a glass!

- 2 inch slice medium size **pineapple**
- ½ mug **coconut milk** (straight from the coconut for preference, otherwise organic/fairtrade from shop)
- ¼ peeled **banana**
- ¼ **mango** (de-stoned)
- 1 handful crushed **ice**

Juice the pineapple and pour into blender. Add the banana, mango, coconut milk and ice. Blend – pour – enjoy!

Smoothie benefits This tropical delight is bursting with potassium – which is important for a healthy nervous system and regular heart rhythm. This mineral alone helps to prevent stroke, aids proper muscle contraction and works with sodium to control the body's water balance. Also rich in vitamins B and C, folic acid, magnesium, 'good' fats, iron and calcium. Coconut milk is also low in calories!

utterly orange

Scrumptious juicy **orange** juice, **blended** with **thick** creamy live **yogurt** and a ripe delicious **banana**

Simply sophisticated and utterly orange.

2 medium, juicy **oranges** (peeled – leaving pith on)
150g low-fat live **yogurt**
½ **banana**
4 **ice cubes** or a small handful **crushed ice**

Juice the oranges and pour into the blender. Add the yogurt, banana and ice into the blender. Blend – pour – enjoy!

Smoothie benefits The orange juice helps to lower blood cholesterol, the friendly bacteria in the yogurt keep a natural balance in the gut and bananas are a natural body cooler. The smoothie is also rich in potassium, vitamin B6, magnesium, natural sugars, amino acids and anti-oxidants.

banana aid

Fresh **banana** blended with delicious extracted **apple** and **lemon** juice and **ice**

This recipe was first made high in the mountains in Turkey on one of my juice retreats. We all had our fill of 'green' juices and just needed something sweet and sustaining. This recipe combines Juice Master's Homemade Sherbet Lemonade with fresh banana to bring you one of the most refreshing, sustaining, tastiest and healthiest smoothies in the book.

2 **apples** (Golden Delicious or Royal Gala if possible)
⅓ **lemon** (with skin on if unwaxed)
1 whole **banana**
1 small handful crushed **ice**

Juice the apple and lemon. Pour into the blender with banana and ice. Blend – pour – enjoy!

Smoothie benefits If you are feeling a little off colour this smoothie is designed to come to your aid. Rich in vitamins A, B1, B2, B6 and C, iron and potassium, the bananas alone can stimulate the production of haemoglobin in the blood and so help in cases of anaemia. Excellent for heartburn since, despite the lemon, this smoothie has a natural antacid effect. It also contains plenty of natural sugars, anti-oxidants and amino acids. And it also tastes amazing – which helps!

natural protein shake

Nature's finest extracted pure **apple** juice, blended with fresh, ripe **banana** and scrummy **blueberries**

This really is Mother Nature's protein power punch. No unnatural 'protein' powders, artificial amino acids or scary steroids are to be found in this protein-packed smoothie. It is bursting with flavour as well as oozing essential amino acids – the body's building blocks for protein.

2 **apples** (Golden Delicious or Royal Gala for preference)
1 handful fresh **blueberries**
½ **banana** (fairtrade if possible)
1 small handful crushed **ice**

Juice the apples. Put the banana, blueberries and ice along with apple juice in the blender. Blend – pour – enjoy!

Smoothie benefits Bananas have four times the protein, twice the carbohydrate, three times the phosphorus, five times the vitamin A and twice the other vitamins and minerals than apples. Not bad when you think that apples are loaded with vitamins A, B2, B3, B6 and C, as well as being one of the most nutritionally rich foods on the planet. Blueberries are one of nature's superfoods and are also loaded with amino acids – the building blocks for protein. A true protein power food.

brazilian superfood smoothie

The gorgeous creamy texture of orange and pineapple juice blended with the tanginess of fresh blueberries

There are foods from nature and then there are superfoods. This smoothie is packed with them.

- 1 inch slice medium size **pineapple**
- 1 large peeled **orange** (peeled but leave the pith on)
- 1 small handful fresh **blueberries**
- 1 small handful crushed **ice**

Juice the pineapple and orange. Place the blueberries, juice and ice into the blender. Blend – pour – enjoy.

Smoothie benefits This divine-tasting smoothie is packed with anti-oxidants and vitamins C and E. These nutritional anti-ageing powerhouses help keep skin soft, clear and elastic.

Juicy boost

For a goji and acai berry boost, simply add 1 heaped teaspoon of Juice Master's Ultimate Berry Boost. These berries will load up this smoothie with even more anti-oxidants, vitamic C and beta-carotene.

banana 'n' honey zest

Creamy **banana** combined with **fresh OJ** and a hint of nature's finest **mouth-watering** Manuka active **honey**

This combination works perfectly together, with the creaminess of the banana and the sweetness of the honey subtly balancing the tanginess of the fresh OJ.

2 juicy **oranges**
½ ripe **banana**
1 teaspoon **Manuka active honey** (or whichever variety you have)
1 small handful **ice**

Peel the oranges, leaving as much of the white pith as possible (as this is where most of the vitamins and nutrients are to be found). Simply juice the oranges and pour into the blender with the banana, honey and ice. Blend – pour – enjoy!

Smoothie benefits Bananas are one of the best sources of potassium, essential for maintaining normal blood pressure and heart function. The banana delivers a perfect source of slow release energy, while the honey gives a much quicker energy fix. If you're a sports enthusiast or looking for a quick pick-me-up, you will love the potassium-power delivered by this high energy smoothie.

mangolicious

Mouth-watering **mango** and succulent **pineapple**, combined with **creamy** live **yogurt**

This recipe is smooth, succulent and scrummy!

½ juicy **mango**
⅓ medium **pineapple**
2 tablespoons low-fat live **yogurt**
1 small handful **ice**

Peel the mango and carefully cut the flesh away from the stone. Wash the pineapple and cut into chunks for juicing. Simply juice the pineapple (with the skin on) and pour into the blender with the mango, yogurt and ice. Blend – pour – enjoy!

Smoothie benefits By combining the flesh of the mango with the yogurt this creates a gorgeous, thick, creamy and filling smoothie. The live yogurt is bursting with friendly bacteria that furnish the intestine and fight bacterial infections as well as aid digestion. The delicious and aromatic mango is a terrific source of potassium and vitamins A and C.

any-berry surprise

As the name suggests, this recipe allows you to use whichever berries are in season, are fresh in your fridge, sat in your freezer or, if you're very lucky, growing in your orchard/hedge! Clearly, depending on which variety you use, the taste will vary and hence the 'surprise'. If you use more than one type of berry you will create a really deep, intense-flavoured smoothie with an unbelievable rich colour.

2 **apples** (Golden Delicious or Royal Gala are best)
1 small handful (each) **raspberries, strawberries, blueberries, blackberries, currants, loganberries** (any or all!)
1 small handful **ice**

Simply wash and juice the apples. Pour the apple juice into the blender, add the berries and ice. Blend – pour – enjoy!

Smoothie benefits Berries are a truly enjoyable way of getting anti-oxidants and phytonutrients into your body. They are well known for their disease-fighting properties and their ability to nourish and enhance the skin. Packed with vitamin C, berries are great for the immune system and contain many anti-cancer properties. They are rich in lutein, which is important for healthy vision, and the darker berries contain powerful anti-oxidants, which may help to slow down the ageing process. These clever little berries benefit the body on the inside as well as the outside!

Simple, gorgeous smoothies

117

pure peachy passion

The soft tender flesh from the ripe peach is perfectly united with the sub-tropical, aromatic flavour of the mysterious passion fruit. This distinctive, unique, fleshy purple fruit has a musky, sweet, yet tart flavour, which is flawlessly balanced by the soft, understated taste of the delicate peach – umm peachy!

2 **apples** (Golden Delicious or Royal Gala are best)
1 ripe **peach**
1 **passion fruit**
1 small handful **ice**

Simply wash and juice the apples. Gently cut the flesh away from the peach and place in the blender. Cut the passion fruit in half and scoop the flesh out into the blender. Add the apple juice and ice. Blend – pour – enjoy!

Smoothie benefits Passion fruit has been the staple diet of people in the Amazon rainforest for eons. South American indigenous tribes believe this unique fruit offers many healing properties and is most notably used as a heart tonic. It is also a great source of vitamins A and C as well as containing high levels of potassium. Vitamin B3 (niacin) found in the peach helps lower cholesterol and improve circulation.

strawberries & cream
(but without the cream!)

Sweet succulent strawberries complemented by thick creamy yogurt and the exquisite complex aroma of the dark, rich, organic vanilla bean, make this smoothie simply divine. This is a mouth-watering yet guilt-free variation on the much-loved great British classic.

1 handful ripe **strawberries**
2 **apples** (Golden Delicious or Royal Gala are best)
½ **vanilla bean** (the raw organic vanilla bean is the ultimate but you can always use a teaspoon of vanilla extract – totally avoid vanilla essence)
3 tablespoons low-fat live **yogurt**
1 small handful **ice**

Simply wash and juice the apples. Remove the stalks from the strawberries, wash and place in the blender. Either cut open half a vanilla bean and scrape out the vanilla pods or add one teaspoon vanilla extract to the blender. Add the live yogurt, apple juice and ice. Blend – pour – enjoy!

Smoothie benefits The major benefit, of course, is that you can satisfy your desire for strawberries and ice cream without the associated creamy calories. Strawberries are abundant in nutrients, minerals, phytonutrients and anti-oxidants. They contain ellagic acid, which has anti-cancer properties as well as the ability to reduce the signs of ageing. The live yogurt is bursting with friendly bacteria that furnish the intestine and fight bacterial infections as well as aiding digestion. Vanilla beans not only taste sensational but are also known for their ability to decrease anxiety and reduce nausea.

pink passion

The vibrant red strawberries, plus the distinctive flavour of the exotic passion fruit and the smooth velvety texture of natural yogurt, are all combined with the bittersweet juice of freshly extracted grapefruit. This creates an almost indescribable experience for your tastebuds to savour.

½ peeled **pink grapefruit** (leave white pith on)
2 **passion fruit**
100g low-fat live **yogurt** (if vegan use soya yogurt)
1 small handful **strawberries**
4 **ice** cubes

Juice the grapefruit. Cut the passion fruit in half, scoop out insides and put into the blender along with strawberries, yogurt and ice. Blend – pour – love your juice!

Smoothie benefits Grapefruits are packed with vitamin C, which helps to sweep up free radical damage and aids the body's absorption of iron and calcium. They also contain salicylic acid, which helps to shift inorganic calcium which may have formed deposits in the cartilage of the joints. This smoothie is rich in calcium, beta-carotene, potassium, natural sugars, amino acids and a tremendous amount of anti-oxidants, which help to slow down the signs of ageing as well as keeping the immune system strong.

cherrylicious

Prepare to experience the dreamy delights of succulent cherries, blended with the natural sweetness of freshly extracted apple juice and accompanied by a generous serving of pure natural live yogurt. This thick, sweet, creamy smoothie is then brought to perfection by the addition of a subtle twist of zesty, vibrant lime juice!

1 **apple** (Golden Delicious or Royal Gala are best)
1 handful **cherries** (de-stoned)
200g low-fat live **yogurt**
1 **lime** (peeled but leave the pith on)
4 **ice cubes** or a small handful **crushed ice**

Juice the apple. Pour the juice in the blender and add the rest of the ingredients. Blend – pour – love your juice!

Smoothie benefits Cherries are one of nature's superfoods. Some varieties contain over 17 natural compounds that work together to promote a healthy body. The 'tart' varieties contain high concentrations of a compound that appears to have the potential to help prevent, stabilize and possibly even eliminate cancer. (According to Raymond Hohl MD, at the University of Iowa, a natural compound found in tart cherries – perillyl alcohol (POH) – 'shuts down the growth of cancer cells by depriving them of the proteins they need to grow.' He went on to say that, 'It works on every kind of cancer we've tested it against.') And that's just this one component. I haven't even mentioned the calcium, vitamins A, B, B1, B2, B6 and C, potassium, anti-oxidants, natural sugars and, and, and …

'nectar of the gods'

Freshly extracted **pineapple** blended with **banana** and the wonderful **nectar** of the delicious **Agave**

In its native home of Mexico, Agave is known as the 'nectar of the gods' and, believe me, this smoothie is nothing short of heavenly!

- ½ medium **pineapple**
- 1 good squirt organic **Agave nectar** (you can get this from most supermarkets – or direct from the Groovy Food company)
- 1 whole **banana** (fairtrade if you can)
- 4 **ice cubes** or a small handful **crushed ice**

Juice the pineapple. Add juice along with everything else to the blender. Blend – pour – love your juice!

Smoothie benefits While regular table sugar has a GI (glycaemic index) value of 68, and honey a GI of 55, the value of Agave nectar is between 11 and 19 – a very low GI. This means that the sweetener is safe for diabetics and, as it's 3 times sweeter than table sugar, you also need to use less. Nectar of the Gods is also rich in vitamins A, B6 and C, folic acid, magnesium, fibre, potassium and iron.

nutty blueberry cream

Smooth, creamy, buttery almonds, combined with decadent blueberries and accompanied by thick live yogurt

This deep vibrant blue opulent smoothie is not only delicious with a capital D but it's also a smoothie you can get your teeth into.

1 **apple** (Royal Gala or Golden Delicious are best)
1 small handful **almonds** (soaked overnight)
150g low-fat live **yogurt** (if vegan use soya yogurt)
1 small handful **blueberries** (fresh or frozen)
4 **ice cubes** or a small handful **crushed ice**

Juice the apple and pour into the blender. Add all the other ingredients. Blend till smooth – pour – love the nuts!

Smoothie benefits High in essential good fats, extremely alkalizing and loaded with anti-oxidants, potassium, vitamins, minerals and amino acids. Almonds are also high in calcium, as well as the banana, making this smoothie an excellent one for healthy bones and teeth.

very seedy mango

Ripe, fleshy **mango** combined with **smooth low-fat live yogurt** and the perfect trio of **pumpkin, sesame** and **sunflower** seeds

The amino-acid-rich seeds not only provide an interesting crunch to this otherwise smooth concoction, but also add a truly satisfactory intensity.

- 1 **apple** (not a Granny Smith)
- 1 small handful **mixed seeds** (pumpkin, sesame, sunflower – you can get good mixed seeds in most supermarkets)
- 150g low-fat live **yogurt** (if vegan use soya yogurt)
- ½ ripe medium **mango**
- 4 **ice cubes** or a small handful **crushed ice**

Juice the apple and pour into blender. Add all other ingredients. Blend – pour – love the seediness of it all!

Smoothie benefits Pumpkin seeds are rich in protein, iron, zinc and phosphorus; 100g pumpkin seeds contain 29g protein, 11.2mg iron and 1144mg phosphorus. Sesame seeds are an excellent source of protein and calcium: 100g sesame seeds contain 26.4g protein, 12.6mg vitamin B3, 7.8mg iron, 131mg calcium and 10.3mg zinc. Sunflower seeds are a good source of potassium and phosphorus: 100g sunflower seeds contain 24g protein and 7.1mg iron and 120mg calcium. That's just the seeds! Add the remainder of the ingredients and you have an extremely healthy smoothie, excellent for the skin and immune system.

new zealand special

Vibrant green **kiwi fruit** and zesty juicy **oranges** all blended together with fresh, ripe, creamy **banana** and sweetened with dreamy delicious native **Manuka active honey**

2 medium juicy **oranges** (peeled but keep pith on)
1 teaspoon **Manuka active honey** (can be bought virtually anywhere)
2 **kiwi fruit** (green or gold, but peeled)
½ medium **banana**
4 **ice cubes** or a handful **crushed ice**

Juice the oranges and pour into blender. Add the rest of the ingredients. Blend until smooth – pour – love the taste of New Zealand!

Smoothie benefits Manuka honey only comes from New Zealand. It is rich in many vitamins and minerals and has incredible antibacterial properties. Kiwi fruit contain twice as much vitamin C as oranges and are rich in calcium, magnesium, phosphorus, potassium and sodium.

yogurt and plum melt

Thick creamy low-fat live yogurt combined with juicy 'melt in the mouth' plums all blended with the finest apple juice

Sometimes the simplest of combinations create the most mouth-watering flavours and this is certainly one of those occasions.

2 medium **apples**
4 **plums** (de-stoned)
150g low-fat live **yogurt**
4 **ice cubes** or a small handful **crushed ice**

Juice the apples and pour into the blender. Add the rest of the ingredients to the blender. Blend until smooth — pour — love the creamy plum texture!

Smoothie benefits Plums are an excellent source of potassium, fibre and vitamins A and C. They are rich in anti-oxidants and also contain the amino acid tryptophan, which is used by the body to produce the neurotransmitter serotonin — the happy brain chemical! The live yogurt will help to maintain a healthy gut and the apple is loaded with B vitamins and the fibre in pectin to sweep your insides clean.

raspberry fizzle

Fresh **raspberries** and **yogurt** blended together with a touch of **fizz** and **ice**

The gentle bubbles of naturally carbonated water adds a subtle fizzle to this juicy raspberry smoothie.

1 large handful **raspberries**
150g low-fat live **yogurt**
100ml mineral **water** (any fizzy mineral water is good but Perrier is best)
4 **ice cubes** or a handful **crushed ice**

No need for your juicer – just your blender! Place all ingredients into the blender. Blend – pour – enjoy the fizzy edge to this sharp smoothie!

Smoothie benefits Raspberries may not be classed in the same superfood bracket as blueberries, acai or goji, but they are still packed with vitamins C and E, calcium, magnesium, phosphorus, sodium, ellagic acid, fibre, zinc, iron and anti-oxidants. This smoothie is excellent for maintaining a proper water balance and blood pH, and it helps good kidney function and is excellent for bones and teeth.

lemon nectar

A truly dreamy **delicious** combination of **pineapple** juice, thick live **yogurt** and the juice of one **whole** citrus fresh **lemon**, drizzled with natural **Agave nectar**

- 1 **lemon** (keep the skin on if unwaxed)
- 1 inch thick slice medium **pineapple** (juice with skin on if your juicer can take it or the fruit is organic)
- 150g low-fat live **yogurt**
- 1 large squirt organic **Agave nectar** (available in most supermarkets and health stores or direct from the Groovy Food company)
- 4 **ice cubes** or a small handful **crushed ice**

Juice the lemon and pineapple and pour into the blender. Add rest of ingredients to blender. Blend – pour – enjoy the lemon lift!

Smoothie benefits The yogurt and low GI sweetener means this smoothie won't cause a sudden spike in your blood sugar levels – meaning it's cool for diabetics (but drink slowly). Loaded with vitamin C, as well as rich in potassium, bromeline and folic acid, it also contains calcium, anti-oxidants, magnesium, phosphorus, beta-carotene and bioflavonoids.

breakfast on the move

This is an alternative to the ever so popular Breakfast on the Go found in our Juice Master Juice 'n' Smoothie bars. You can use any berries you like but the combination of strawberries and raspberries works particularly well.

1 handful fresh **strawberries**
1 handful fresh **raspberries**
150g low-fat live **yogurt**
150g **soya milk**
50g **muesli** (no added sugar/salt)
A small handful **ice cubes**

Place all the ingredients in the blender. Blend — enjoy!

Smoothie benefits If your usual breakfast is a couple of slices of white, nutrient-devoid toast with full-fat butter and sugar-loaded jam, then your body and waistline are in for a real treat. Replacing your regular breakfast with this delicious alternative will not only cut out the fat and artificial sugar, but will also supply the body with a huge dollop of goodness. The raspberries and strawberries contain a distinguished array of vitamins, minerals and anti-oxidants that boost the immune system as well as destroy free radical damage. The friendly bacteria found in the low-fat live yogurt furnishes the intestine with 'good' bacteria to aid digestion and fight bad bacterial infections. Muesli provides a great source of dietary fibre, minerals, vitamins and natural sugar. This smoothie is bursting with goodness and will certainly keep you filled up till lunchtime!

berry beauty

Deep, **dark**, mysterious **blueberries** and **blackberries**, carefully combined with the freshly extracted juice of **two** sweet **apples** and a **generous** helping of creamy live **yogurt**

The rich colour and intensity of the berries combined with the smooth, silky texture of the yogurt make this smoothie utterly delicious.

2 **apples** (Golden Delicious or Royal Gala are best)
1 handful **blueberries**
1 handful **blackberries**
200g low-fat live **yogurt**
1 handful **ice** cubes

Juice the apples. Put the blueberries, blackberries, yogurt and ice into the blender with the apple juice. Blend – pour – enjoy!

Smoothie benefits The berries are bursting with anti-oxidants, vitamins B, C, E and K, calcium, iron, magnesium and phosphorus. What's more, they contain ellagic acid, which is an anti-ageing phytochemical that is believed to slow down the signs of ageing. So this really is a very berry beauty!

cool twist

Pale **green** succulent **grapes** straight from the vine, combined with the cool taste of fresh **kiwi fruit**, a hint of **apple**, a twist of **lime** and a dollop of fresh live **yogurt**

Cool, refreshing and utterly delicious!

2 **apples** (Golden Delicious or Royal Gala are best)
½ **lime** (peeled but leave pith on)
1 small bunch of **grapes**
1 **kiwi fruit** (peeled)
200g low-fat live **yogurt**
1 handful **ice** cubes

Juice the apples and lime. Put the grapes, kiwi fruit flesh, yogurt and ice into the blender. Blend – pour – savour this delicious flavour!

Smoothie benefits Grape juice is believed to lower the chances of blood clots in the heart as well as calming the nervous system. It has a high mineral content that helps to strengthen the alkaline reserves in the body; it promotes good bowel movement, proper kidney function and regulates the heart beat. That's just the grape juice! You add the rest of the ingredients and you have – vitamins A, B, B2, B3, B6, C and E, magnesium, potassium and many more minerals and anti-oxidants – and just think of the benefits!

Simple, gorgeous smoothies

cherry tart

Cherries and ice blended with freshly extracted orange juice

This smoothie is vibrant, tangy and a little bit tart. If thick creamy yogurt isn't your thing and you're more about the zesty flavour of fresh OJ and the slightly tangy taste of cherries, this simple yet seriously good smoothie is the one for you.

2 medium **oranges** (fairtrade where possible)
1 small handful **cherries**
4 **ice cubes** or a small handful **crushed ice**

Peel the oranges, keeping as much of the pith as possible (this is where most of the nutrients and flavonoids are to be found) and then juice. Remove the stalks and stones from the cherries and add to the blender. Add the orange juice and ice to the blender. Blend – pour – enjoy!

Smoothie benefits According to researchers from Michigan State University, anthocyanins – the red pigments in cherries – are used to reduce inflammation of the joints in certain prescription drugs. There is lab evidence which shows that drinking a glass of cherry juice may be more effective than aspirin. It has also been reported that cherry juice therapy reduces the pain of arthritis, gout and headaches. This smoothie is loaded with vitamins, minerals, anti-oxidants, natural sugars and amino acids.

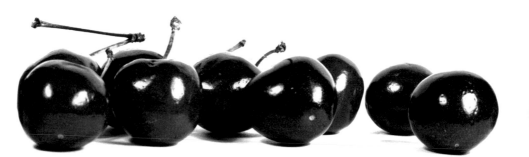

salad smoothie

Rich **avocado**, accompanied by **water-rich cucumber**, sodium-rich **celery**, apple, sweet **baby leaf spinach** and **watercress**

We don't always get around to eating enough salads, so it's nice to know you can always drink one!

2 **apples** (Golden Delicious or Royal Gala are best)
1 inch chunk medium **cucumber**
½ stick **celery**
1 generous handful **baby leaf spinach**
1 small handful **watercress**
½ ripe **avocado** (organic if possible)
4 **ice cubes** or a small handful **crushed ice**

Juice the apples, cucumber, celery, spinach and watercress. Add the flesh of the avocado to the blender along with the juice and ice. Blend — pour — marvel at the miracle that is salad in a glass!

Smoothie benefits It is thought that avocados are the only food on the planet which you could live on exclusively. They contain essential fats, natural sugars, amino acids (nature's body builders), vitamins, minerals, organic water and enzymes. Spinach juice is rich in nature's liquid sunshine — chlorophyll — as well as beta-carotene, folic acid, iron, choline and vitamins A, C and E. Add the rest of the ingredients and you have all the goodness of a salad, but in a liquid form.

savoury sweet

Rich, creamy organic **avocado** combined with the sweet taste of **freshly** extracted **apple juice** and zesty natural **lime** juice

2 **apples** (Golden Delicious or Royal Gala are best)
½ peeled **lime** (leave as much pith as possible)
½ ripe **avocado** (organic if possible)
4 **ice cubes** or a small handful **crushed ice**

Juice the apples and lime. Add the flesh of the avocado to the blender along with the juice and ice. Blend – pour – enjoy!

Smoothie benefits Savoury Sweet contains vitamins A, B, B1, B2, B3, B6, C, E and K, folic acid, calcium, potassium, bioflavonoids, iron, magnesium, manganese, phosphorus, zinc, essential fats, pectin, malic acid, natural sugars and anti-oxidants. This smoothie will help alkaline the system, clean the colon and regulate the heart.

swamp juice

Perhaps not the best name in the world — but, hey, it looks like swamp juice! However, don't let that put you off; looks are often deceiving and this swampy looking drink tastes amazing. It is incredibly creamy and has a wonderful head on it.

2 **apples** (Golden Delicious or Royal Gala are best)
½ stick **celery**
½ **carrot** (organic)
1 tiny chunk **courgette**
1 small handful **baby leaf spinach**
1 small handful **kale**
1 very, very small handful **parsley** (it's pretty potent)
1 small handful **alfalfa spouts** (not always easy to get, so maybe leave out)
¼ **lemon** (peeled)
½ **avocado** (organic if possible)
1 handful **ice**

Juice all the produce the except the avocado. Add the flesh of the avocado to the blender along with the juice and ice. Blend — pour —and enjoy how very, very good this is for your body!

Smoothie benefits Packed with just about every vitamin and mineral known to wo/mankind — there are just far, far too many to mention — when you look at all the ingredients that are going into this smoothie you intuitively know it's extremely wonderful for you!

fruit 'n' nut case

Freshly extracted apple juice combined with mixed nuts, mixed fruit and yogurt

This should satisfy the desires of even the most diehard fruit and nut heads. This is a smoothie that you can actually get your teeth into. The trick is not to blend it for too long — that way you can still enjoy chewing on the occasional nut or juicy raisin.

2 **apples** (Royal Gala or Golden Delicious are best)
1 small handful **almonds** (soaked overnight)
1 small handful **brazil nuts**
1 small handful **cashews**
1 small handful **raisins**
1 small handful **mixed frozen fruit**
2 tablespoons low-fat live **yogurt**

Juice the apples and pour into the blender. Add the nuts, raisins, mixed fruit and yogurt to the blender. Blend quickly — pour —and enjoy!

Smoothie benefits Loaded with zinc, selenium, essential fats, protein and calcium. Raisins are rich in natural sugars and vitamins and the live yogurt will help replace friendly bacteria in the gut and slow the absorption of sugars in the bloodstream. It also contains vitamins A, B1, B2, B6 and C, beta-carotene, iron, magnesium, phosphorus, potassium, sulphur, pectin and malic acid.

peachy apricot nectar

The sublime flavour of **peach**, **apricot** and **nectarine**, delicately **blended** with rich, creamy **pineapple** and deep, dark **Manuka** active **honey**

½ medium **pineapple**
1 **peach** (de-stoned)
1 **apricot** (de-stoned)
1 **nectarine** (de-stoned)
1 good dollop **Manuka active honey** (any honey will do but Manuka is best)
1 small handful **ice**

Juice the pineapple and pour into the blender. Add the flesh of the peach, apricot and nectarine, honey and ice. Blend – pour –and enjoy!

Smoothie benefits Rich in potassium and vitamin C, this gorgeous smoothie has excellent antibacterial properties and is great for the skin. Like all the smoothies in this book it is loaded with anti-oxidants, helping to defy the signs of ageing as well as maintaining a good heath defence system. It also contains calcium, magnesium, iron, natural sugars, amino acids, phytonutrients and nature's finest organic natural water – direct from the fruits!

Simple, gorgeous smoothies

cranberry 'n' orange

Freshly extracted orange juice blended with cranberries, bananas and ice

Cranberries have an instantly refreshing flavour that beautifully complements the zestiness of freshly extracted orange juice. This perfect partnership, combined with creamy puréed banana and crushed ice, means this smoothie is as refreshing as it is delicious!

2 medium **oranges** (peeled – leave as much of pith on as possible)
1 small handful **cranberries** (fresh or frozen)
½ **banana** (fairtrade if possible)
4 **ice cubes** or a small handful **crushed ice**

Juice the oranges and add to the blender. Add the cranberries, banana and ice. Blend – pour –and enjoy!

Smoothie benefits Cranberry juice contains something called quininic acid, better known as quinine. Quininic acid is so powerful that it converts to another acid that helps to lift toxins not only from the bladder and kidneys but also from the prostate and testicles. Cranberries also have vitamins A and C, iodine, calcium, beta-carotene, folic acid, magnesium, phosphorus and potassium in them.

lemon, ginger 'n' banana blast

Freshly extracted apple, lemon and ginger juice blended with banana and ice

This is a twist on the Lemon Ginger Zinger which is a huge hit in our Juice Master Juice 'n' Smoothie Bars. I have turned this popular juice into a scrumptious smoothie by removing the carrot and instead adding some gorgeous ripe banana. The sharpness of the ginger is balanced beautifully by the soft puréed banana – this twist on the original is an absolute winner!

2 **apples** (Golden Delicious or Royal Gala are best)
⅓ **lemon** (keep skin on if unwaxed)
1 inch piece fresh **ginger** (with skin on)
1 **banana** (fairtrade where possible)
4 **ice cubes** or a small handful **crushed ice**

Juice the apple, lemon and ginger and pour into the blender. Add the banana and ice. Blend – pour – enjoy!

Smoothie benefits This smoothie is loaded with potassium, natural antibiotics, B vitamins, vitamin C, natural sugars, amino acids, anti-oxidants, natural water, magnesium, pectin and much, much more …

just juice

pure liquid gold

no artificial sugar
no artificial fat
no artificial colours
no artificial flavours
no preservatives
no sweeteners
no additives
no stabilisers
and

no guilt ... after all, nobody has ever had a
freshly extracted juice and thought, 'Oh I
wish I hadn't done that!'

There are juices and then there are freshly-extracted, make-your-taste-buds-dance-for-joy juices. The following recipes have been carefully designed with taste and health in mind. Whoever said that if it tastes good, it can't be good for you, clearly either never juiced, or just didn't know what they were doing.

This tantalizing selection of freshly extracted juices is superb for your mind and excellent for your body. As every juice deposits some liquid gold into your health bank account, your internal bank manager will be one happy healthy camper!

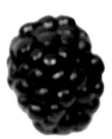

sweet carrot 'n' apple pie

Freshly extracted **carrot** and **apple** juice with a pinch of **cinnamon**

Think of a slice of Momma's apple pie and you have an idea of what this extremely creamy juice tastes like. Carrot juice is surprisingly sweet and mixes extremely well with freshly extracted apple juice. Once you add just a little pinch of cinnamon, you turn a simple apple and carrot juice into a creamy, rich drink which tastes like pie!

1 **carrot**
2 **apples**
1 very small handful crushed **ice**
1 pinch powdered **cinnamon**

Juice the apples and carrot. Pour into a glass with ice. Add pinch of cinnamon. Savour in the mouth — tastes like apple and carrot pie.

Juicy benefits Carrots are the beta-carotene kings of the veg world and beta-carotene (pro-vitamin A) is regarded as the best cancer preventative in the world. Carrot juice also contains vitamins B, C, E and K as well as calcium, iron, magnesium, potassium and folic acid. Add the apple juice and you've just added malic acid (which helps to remove impurities), pectin (a great source of soluble fibre), phosphorus and sulphur.

green super fuel

The freshly extracted juice from crisp Golden Delicious apples, mixed with the chlorophyll-rich powerful juice of baby leaf spinach and courgette, finished off with the zesty kick of fresh lime – all poured over ice

2 apples (Golden Delicious)
1 large handful baby leaf spinach (or what you can get)
1 inch slice courgette
1 lime (peeled , but leave pith on)
1 small handful crushed ice

Place one apple in a wide chute juicer without turning on the machine. Pack in the spinach, courgette and lime and 'sandwich' this with the other apple. Push through, pour over ice and feel the power of the green super fuel.

Juicy benefits Courgette (or zucchini) is rich in potassium, vitamin A and phosphorus. Phosphorus is required for blood clotting, good bone and teeth formation and helps with kidney function. The juice also contains vitamins B, B1, B2, B3, B6, C and E, chlorophyll, folic acid, iron, calcium, magnesium, natural sugars, malic acid, soluble fibre and nature's finest organic water.

sunny de'bright

Vitamin-rich **creamy** juice from **Florida oranges**, with the **sweetness** of fresh **apple juice** and the added **sunshine** zing of fresh **lime** juice — all **poured** over crushed **ice**

The taste of sunshine in a glass! The name may sound like a famous bottled fruit juice (and I use the word 'fruit' as lightly as I possibly can in relation to that product!) but the texture, taste and health benefits are worlds apart.

2 juicy **Florida oranges** (peeled but with the pith on)
1 **apple** (Golden Delicious or anything but Granny Smiths!)
1 **lime** (peeled with pith on)
1 small handful **crushed ice** or 3 **ice cubes**

Juice the oranges, apple and lime. Pour over ice. Enjoy.

Juicy benefits Just by looking at the ingredients you have probably guessed that this juice is brimming with vitamin C. Vitamin C is an anti-oxidant required for tissue growth and repair, adrenal gland function and healthy gums. This super-vitamin also helps to increase the activity of white blood cells, which are vital for fighting infections and for the immune system. And I haven't even mentioned what the vitamins A, B1, B2 and B6, iron, magnesium, potassium, sulphur, calcium, pectin or malic acid can do!

royal raspberry

Fresh deep rich **raspberries**, sandwiched between succulent **Royal Gala apples**, all pushed through your **juicer** to bring you a sweet, sharp, creamy rich nutrient-packed juice

2 **apples** (Royal Gala, organic if possible)
1 large handful fresh **raspberries**
1 small handful **crushed ice** or 3 **ice cubes**

Without turning the machine on, place one apple in your whole fruit juicer, pack the raspberries in and finish with the other apple. Juice the lot. Pour over ice and LOVE your juice.

Juicy benefits Raspberries are rich in potassium, niacin, zinc, iron, vitamin C and ellagic acid. Like all berries the anti-oxidant levels are high, helping to slow down the signs of ageing and mop up free radical damage. The overall juice also contains vitamin A, most of the B vitamins, calcium, magnesium, phosphorus, sulphur, malic acid, soluble fibre in the form of pectin, natural sugars, natural fats and nature's finest organic water.

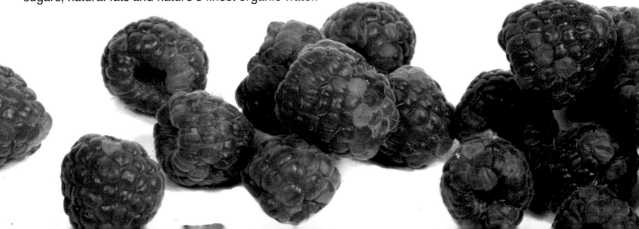

pineapple cream

Fresh **pineapple** juice is the **creamiest** juice in the world by **far** and **occasionally** no other **fruit** or **veg** needs to be added

This is one such occasion. When you juice pineapple you will notice it produces a wonderful pale yellow colour and an incredible head of foam. Although this is 'just' pineapple juice, once you taste it and read the benefits you will see there is no 'just' when it comes to this – my personal favourite – mono juice.

1 medium **pineapple**
1 handful **crushed ice** or 4 **ice cubes**

Juice the pineapple. (You can leave the skin on if your juicer can take it and if the fruit is organic. If it's not organic, just wash and it can still be juiced with the skin on. If you want it really creamy, remove the skin.) Pour over ice – enjoy!

Juicy benefits Pineapples are an excellent source of vitamin C, folic acid, potassium and bromeline. Bromeline is a powerful enzyme that encourages the secretion of hydrochloric acid, which helps to digest protein. The high potassium content is good for healthy muscles and the nervous system, helps to prevent stokes, regulates the transfer of nutrients through cell membranes and is needed to maintain the body's balance of sodium and potassium – an imbalance can lead to heart attacks.

dr juice

A cloudy red juice combining the **sweet** and creamy flavours of freshly extracted **apple** and **carrot** juice with the savoury **sodium** of **celery** and the kick of **lemon** and **ginger**

1 inch slice large **carrot**
2 **apples** (Golden Delicious or Royal Gala are best)
½ stick **celery**
1 small whole raw **beetroot**
½ inch slice unwaxed **lemon**
½ slice **ginger**
ice

Juice the lot, except for the ice. Pour over ice.

Juicy benefits There aren't too many medications your average Dr would give out that contain the array of health-building constituents of Dr Juice. Contains vitamins A, B1, B2, B3, B6, C, E and K, beta-carotene, calcium, iron, magnesium, manganese, phosphorus, potassium, sodium, zinc, folic acid, malic acid, soluble fibre, natural sugars, natural fats, organic natural water and an amazing amount of anti-oxidants. Each vitamin or mineral plays a role in maintaining the overall health of the body and the anti-oxidants will mop up free radical damage caused by fast foods, cigarette smoke, stress and other factors.

juice master's sherbet fennelade

This is an aniseed version of my homemade Sherbet Lemonade and I feel it's even tastier – if that's at all possible. If you think of the days when you used to dip a strand of liquorice into some powdered sherbet, you have pretty much imagined the taste of this freshly made juice. If you aren't a lover of aniseed then you won't much care for this, but if you do LOVE the taste of sherbet-dipped liquorice but don't want the refined sugar and other rubbish, look no further than this taste sensation.

1 generous slice **fennel**
2 **apples** (Golden Delicious)
1 inch slice **lemon** (keep skin on if unwaxed)
1 small handful **crushed ice** or 3 **ice cubes**

Juice the lot, except for the ice. (If you have a whole fruit juicer then place one apple in first – without turning on the machine – add the fennel and lemon and finish with the other apple. Turn on and push through.) Pour over ice – delicious!

Juicy benefits Fennel is a good source of niacin (vitamin B3), calcium, iron, magnesium, phosphorus, copper, folic acid, potassium and manganese. This juice provides about 15 per cent of the vitamin C required daily. The sugars from fennel are released slowly into the body, making it ideal for helping to maintain and manage a healthy weight. This super-juice also contains vitamin A and most of the B vitamins, as well as malic acid and pectin.

pure berry nectar

This wonderful rich-flavoured and bursting with colour juice contains nothing except a selection of nature's finest berries. The combination of fresh blueberry, blackberry, raspberry and strawberry juice poured over some crushed ice provides one of the most delightful and refreshing juices you will ever have the good fortune to taste.

Bursting with nature's finest colours and brimming with anti-ageing anti-oxidants, this juice is about as pure and beneficial as it gets, but, unlike a lot of things that are good for us, this tastes like nectar.

1 handful each of **blueberries**, **strawberries**, **raspberries** and **blackberries**
4 **ice cubes** or a small handful **crushed ice**

Without turning on your whole fruit juicer, pack all of the berries in the chute. Turn on machine on the lower speed and push through slowly. The amount of berries you need is one whole chute worth (if you have Juice Master's Whole Fruit Pro juicer). If you don't have a whole fruit juicer, still pack your chute with berries and juice, and then repeat until all the berries are juiced. Pour into a glass over ice.

Juicy benefits It is almost hard to list all what nature's berries can do as it's a book itself. However, you need to know these berries are nature's most powerful age-defying fruits and are low in calories, have no cholesterol and are loaded with anti-oxidants. The juice contains vitamins C and E, calcium, iron, magnesium, niacin, potassium, phosphorus, sodium, sulphur, beta-carotene, ellagic acid and folic acid.

liquid lunch 'pick-me-up'

If you tend to 'slump' after lunch, try replacing the usual sandwich and crisps or coffee and muffin with this lunchtime 'pick-me-up'. The freshly extracted juice from crisp Golden Delicious apples, mixed with creamy organic carrot juice and zingy lime — topped with some fresh mint — will have you bouncing around in no time.

2 **apples** (Golden Delicious)
1 **carrot** (organic)
1 **lime** (peeled, but leave the pith on)
1 pinch finely chopped **mint**
4 **ice cubes** or a small handful **crushed ice**

Juice everything except the mint and ice. Pour juice into a glass over ice and sprinkle the mint on top. Drink slowly and enjoy.

Juicy benefits The array of natural sugars in it is what gives this juice its 'pick me up' properties, while the anti-oxidants help to mop up any free radical damage which may be occurring due to stress at work. This juice helps to calm the nervous system, provides all of the essential vitamins and minerals required by the body and helps to re-hydrate the system by way of nature's organic natural water contained within all fruits and vegetables.

cool as a ...

No prizes for guessing that this recipe has cucumber in it. Cucumber juice doesn't usually win any awards on the taste front, but when you mix this cooling juice with the sweet, rich juice of freshly extracted apple, lemon and lime, it complements the juice beautifully by toning down the sharpness of the citrus juices and adding its own subtle texture and flavour, without it being overpowering.

⅓ medium **cucumber**
2 **apples** (Royal Gala or Golden Delicious – or anything but Granny Smiths)
1 inch slice unwaxed **lemon**
1 **lime** (peeled, but leave pith on)
3 **ice cubes** or a small handful **crushed ice**

Juice everything except the ice. Pour juice over ice in a glass.

Juicy benefits Cucumbers are renowned for their ability to cool the inner sanctuary of the body. This juice contains vitamins A, B1, B2, B3, B5, B6 and C, beta-carotene, calcium, iron, magnesium, phosphorus, potassium, sulphur, malic acid, pectin, bioflavonoids and folic acid. It's great for cleansing the liver and kidneys, excellent for the hair, nails and skin and a brilliant natural diuretic.

the x factor

A gorgeous, nutrient-packed combination of freshly extracted pineapple and pear juice

All juicy recipes made with nature's finest liquid fuel have the X Factor; however, this pure juice recipe really does have that something extra.

¼ medium **pineapple**
2 **pears** (Conference for preference)
3 **ice cubes** or a small handful **crushed ice**

Juice the pineapple and pear. Pour the juice into a glass over ice.

Juicy benefits Pineapple is rich in vitamin C, potassium, bromeline and folic acid, whilst pear juice is also rich in potassium and vitamin C, as well as many other vitamins and minerals.

Juicy boost

To give this juice even more X factor, add 1 level teaspoon of Juice Master's Ultimate Berry Boost. Its age-defying acai berries contain oleic acids, which help omega-3 essential fats penetrate cell membranes and reduce inflamation — essential for anti-ageing.

on the grapevine

This pure **grape** juice **combines** the deep rich flavour of **red grapes** with the **fresh** feel of the **green** variety

Not all grape juice needs to be fermented and corked – sometimes it just comes fresh from the grape and is drunk there and then. Freshly extracted grape juice is not one that many people try as they tend to simply eat grapes, but the taste of this juice is just so light and refreshing – and so extraordinarily good for such a simple juice – that I can almost guarantee it becomes a part of your regular juicy lifestyle.

1 large handful **red grapes** (ideally taken straight off a vine)
1 large handful **green grapes** (ideally taken straight off a vine)
3 **ice cubes** or a small handful **crushed ice**

Pack the grapes into the chute of the juicer. Turn on machine and push through. Pour over ice and drink slowly.

Juicy benefits When you hear that 'red wine is good for the heart' or that wine in general is 'full of anti-oxidants', it is grape juice, of course, that is being referred to. In its non-fermented form there are more active anti-oxidants than in the 'made into wine' variety. Anti-oxidants are important for mopping up free radical damage, slowing down the ageing process and helping to keep a good 'disease defence system'.

Just juice

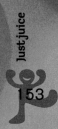

summer breeze

A **sumptuous** mix of **freshly** extracted **mango** and **strawberry** juice over **ice**

It is hard even to say the words 'fresh mango' and 'fresh strawberries' without thinking of summer or, indeed, without your mouth watering. Mango juice is wonderfully thick – almost like treacle – but once diluted with freshly extracted strawberry juice you have the perfect consistency. Once this juice hits your lips you will taste summer.

½ **mango** (ripe and de-stoned)
1 large handful **strawberries**
3 **ice cubes** or a small handful **crushed ice**

Without turning on your juicer, pack the mango into the chute first and then fill your whole fruit juicer with strawberries. Turn on the machine and push through slowly on the slower setting. Pour over ice, sit back, put your feet up and feel the summer breeze!

Juicy benefits Rich in many vitamins and minerals but the ones which come out top in this summer juice are vitamin C, carotenes, potassium, flavonoids and zinc. One strawberry has more vitamin C than one orange, and has 20 per cent of your daily requirement of folic acid (proven to reduce birth defects). This has no cholesterol, an amazing amount of anti-oxidants, natural sugars and a very long list of health benefits.

simply cantaloupe

Like an angel **dancing** on your **tongue** – there's almost **no other way** to describe **pure, sweet, creamy,** mind-blowing **freshly** extracted **Cantaloupe melon** juice

You can juice Cantaloupe melon with the skin on. Yes, simply cut a large slice and juice it! You can't really get more simple than that, and as the vast majority of the nutrients are to be found either just beneath the skin or in the skin itself, your body will be glad of the fact this fruit can be juiced skin and all.

1 large slice **Cantaloupe melon** (wash skin)
3 **ice cubes** or a small handful **crushed ice**

Just juice it! Pour over ice and let the sweet melon nectar sit in your mouth for a short while to savour the flavour.

Juicy benefits An amazing source of vitamins A and C. One glass of Cantaloupe juice is just an average of 56 calories, but provides 103.2 per cent of the daily value for vitamin A. While vitamin A is a fat-soluble anti-oxidant, vitamin C functions as an anti-oxidant in the water-soluble areas of the body. This means that between Cantaloupe's beta-carotene (pro-vitamin A) and vitamin C content, it has all areas covered against damage from harmful free radicals. Vitamin C is also essential for good immune function; it stimulates white cells to fight infection, directly kills many bacteria and viruses and regenerates vitamin E after it has been de-activated by free radicals.

boost juice

If you are in Australia reading this book, the name Boost Juice will mean more to you as a juice bar chain than a recipe. Janine Allis (owner and founder) of Boost Juice — the biggest and most successful juice bar chain in the southern hemisphere — has done an enormous amount in bringing juices and smoothies to the public at large. However, this is not a juice bar chain; it's just a juice, but a juice with an extremely powerful boost.

1 **carrot**
2 **apples**
1 inch slice **lemon** (keep the skin on if unwaxed)
1 **lime** (peeled but leave pith on)
3 **ice cubes** or a small handful **crushed ice**

Juice the lot (except the ice). Pour juice into a glass over ice and feel the boost!

Juicy benefits Rich in beta-carotene (anti-cancer king of the fruit and veg world) as well as nearly all the B vitamins, vitamin C, calcium and magnesium.

Juicy boost

To get this juice to pack an extra punch, add 1 level teaspoon of Juice Master's Ultimate Juice Boost.

christmas in a glass!

No, this isn't juiced turkey! It's a wonderfully 'earthy' juice which combines some of the vegetables most commonly found at the Christmas dinner table. If you are thinking Brussels sprouts, parsnip, cauliflower, carrot, potato, spinach and peas, then you are almost there. I grant the sound of this juice might have even the most regular juicer thinking more than twice before making it, but I have delicately divided the ingredients so that, once mixed with a little sweet freshly extracted apple juice, it tastes pretty damn good. And unlike the veggies at Christmas, these are all very much raw and bursting with nature's natural colours and enzymes.

1 **Brussels sprout**
1 inch chunk **parsnip**
1 **carrot**
1 small **new potato**
1 large handful **spinach**
1 dozen **peas**
1 **cauliflower** floret
2 **apples**
3 **ice cubes** or a small handful **crushed ice**

Juice the lot, except the ice. Pour over the ice – enjoy!

Juicy benefits You only need to look at the ingredients to know that it's good for your health beyond belief. Brussels sprouts contain the potent anti-cancer compound sinigrin, which 'persuades' pre-cancerous cells to commit suicide (a natural process called apoptosis). Add the other ingredients and you have just about every vitamin, mineral and phytonutrient know to wo/mankind.

cranberry, apple & pineapple

Sweet meets tart with this perfect juice combination of cranberry, apple and pineapple

Cranberry juice on its own is far too tart and acidic to drink, but once combined with the sweet, incredibly creamy juice of pineapple and apple, it not only becomes palatable but adds a wonderful kick, and its acidity is reduced greatly.

1 small handful **cranberries** (fresh or frozen)
2 **apples** (Royal Gala or Golden Delicious)
1 inch slice medium **pineapple** (fairtrade if possible)
3 **ice cubes** or a small handful **crushed ice**

Juice the fruit. Pour in a glass over ice. Enjoy.

Juicy benefits Cranberry juice has been used by juice therapists for many, many years to treat liver, kidney and bladder disorders and is excellent for skin conditions such as psoriasis. This juicy combination of ingredients is rich in vitamins A and C, calcium, potassium, iron, quinine, magnesium, malic acid, pectin, natural sugars, nature's natural organic water direct from the fruits, amino acids and anti-oxidants.

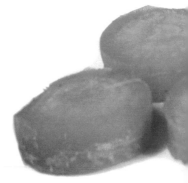

carrot 'n' orange

The **creamy sweet** texture of fresh **carrot** juice mixed with the **vibrant** 'alive' taste of **orange**

Ideally you shouldn't really mix fruit juices with vegetable juices. Apple, pineapple, lemon and lime are the exceptions to this rule, so normally I wouldn't advise orange with a vegetable like carrot. However, this is an exception that proves the rule, as this works incredibly well on the taste front.

1 large **carrot**
1 large juicy **orange** (peeled but leave the pith on)
3 **ice cubes** or a small handful **crushed ice**

Juice the carrot and orange. Pour into a glass over the ice — beautiful!

Juicy benefits High in beta-carotene (pro-vitamin A) as well as vitamins B, C, E and even K; rich in folic acid, magnesium, potassium, iron and calcium. This juice has a cleansing effect on the liver and digestive system and helps to lower blood cholesterol as well. It also aids eye and skin problems.

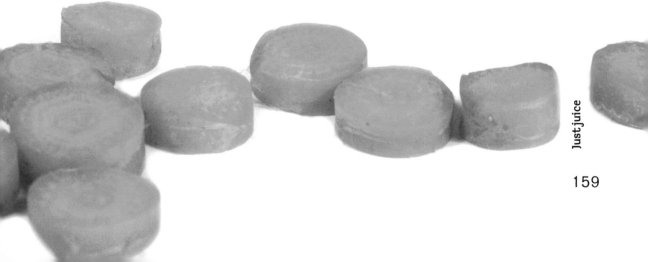

tangerine
ginger zinger

Exquisite tangerine, lemon and ginger juice over ice

This is a take on our Lemon Ginger Zinger which is served all over the country at Juice Master Juice 'n' Smoothie bars. Instead of carrot, we have the surprisingly gorgeous tangerine juice, and I have left out the apple juice here so as not to overwhelm the tangerine flavour. There aren't too many people who have tasted this juice by itself (which over ice is wonderful), let alone had the ginger zinger experience. When in season tangerines are easy to peel, making this juice extremely quick to make.

3 **tangerines** (peeled)
⅓ unwaxed **lemon** (peeled)
½ piece **ginger** (with skin on)
3 **ice cubes** or a small handful **crushed ice**

Juice everything except the ice. Pour juice into a glass over the ice and prepare to be zinged!

Juicy benefits Incredibly rich in vitamin C as well as beta-carotene, calcium, magnesium and potassium. The ginger adds some natural antibiotic properties to this juice and the lemon helps to cleanse the liver and kidneys, as well as contributing some powerful anti-oxidants.

fennel veggie heaven

A beautiful combination of creamy apple juice, cool cucumber, earthy broccoli, zingy lime and aniseed-flavoured fennel

Fennel juice adds such a wonderful flavour to a juice as well as being surprisingly good for you. Despite its vegetable look, fennel is in fact a herb and a powerful one at that, which is why we only use a little bit in the recipe.

¼ small cucumber
3 broccoli florets
1 inch square piece fennel (or equivalent sized slice)
2 apples (Royal Gala or Golden Delicious)
1 lime (peeled, but leave pith on)
3 ice cubes or a small handful crushed ice

Juice everything except the ice. Pour into a glass over ice – love your juice!

Juicy benefits Fennel has twice the vitamin C of an orange and almost as much calcium as whole milk. Unlike milk, most of the calcium is bio-available to the cells, meaning it is better for calcium intake than milk. Fennel can be useful for indigestion and spasm of the digestive tract. It is an anti-carcinogenic herb and helps to calm the nervous system. Broccoli is one of the few fruits or vegetables on the planet that contain both vitamins A and K. Vitamin K is essential for the prevention of osteoporosis.

summer crush

The pure juice of intense **blueberries**, vibrant **raspberries** and delicious **strawberries** combined with **freshly** extracted **apple** juice and poured over crushed **ice**

2 **apples** (Golden Delicious or Royal Gala)
1 handful fresh **blueberries**
1 handful fresh **raspberries**
1 handful fresh **strawberries**

If you have a whole fruit juicer then this is sooo easy; if not, follow the same method but you will need to cut up the apple first. Place one apple in the chute of the juicer. Add the berries and then the second apple. Juice – pour over crushed ice – enjoy!

Juicy benefits This combination of berries contains a phenomenal number of vital vitamins and minerals. The juice is also bursting with folic acid and anti-oxidants, which are excellent for the immune system as well as in the fight against free radical damage.

non-alcoholic rosé

Delicious white **grapes** straight from the vineyard, rich, full-bodied, crisp **Royal Gala apples**, enriched with the **pink** tones and hearty flavour of fresh juicy **raspberries**

This is an excellent, non-alcoholic alternative to traditional Rosé. Enjoy over an afternoon lunch with the added pleasure of no mid-afternoon alcohol slump.

2 **apples** (Royal Gala)
1 small bunch **white grapes**
1 small handful **raspberries**
100ml **mineral water** (Perrier is best)

Place one apple in the chute of the juicer. Add the grapes, berries and the second apple. Juice — pour into a glass — add the mineral water. Cheers!

Juicy benefits a) No hangover! b) By replacing wine with this non-alcoholic version your skin and liver will love you. Instead of dehydrating your cells and skin with gone-off, fermented fruit you will furnish your body with live, high water content, vitamin-packed freshly extracted fruit juice.

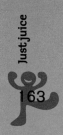

peachy pineapple zest

The freshly extracted juice of divine **peaches**, zesty **nectarines** and rich creamy **pineapple**, combined together and poured over crushed **ice** create something quite **magical**

2 **peaches** (de-stoned)
2 **nectarines** (de-stoned)
⅓ medium **pineapple** (with skin on)
1 small handful crushed **ice**

Place the peaches, nectarine and pineapple in the juicer. Juice – pour over the ice – enjoy!

Juicy benefits It's common knowledge that all citrus fruit are a great source of vitamin C, however you might be surprised to learn that so are peaches. Vitamin C is required for tissue growth and repair as well as being very important in fighting infections and boosting the immune system. This juice is also rich in vitamin A, so this zesty juice is excellent for the skin and eyes.

orange juice
with a twist

This isn't just **orange** juice; this is the **freshly** extracted juice of the **ripest**, juiciest, **Sicilian oranges** enriched with a twist of **lime**

3 **oranges** (peeled; Sicilian sound sexy, but in reality any will do!)
½ **lime** (peeled)
1 small handful crushed **ice**

Place the oranges and lime in the juicer. Juice – pour over the ice – enjoy!

Juicy benefits Oranges are a famous source of vitamin C, but they are particularly powerful at cleaning the intestinal tract of bacteria and toxins, too. Oranges and limes contain citric acid, which is the most powerful fruit acid. This juice, therefore, is very good at eliminating toxins from the system and cleaning the liver and kidneys.

parsnip refresher

Freshly extracted apple, parsnip and mint juice over ice

This is one of those times when the proof of the pudding is in the tasting. The ingredients may sound a little strange, but the combination really works. It's fresh, it's invigorating and, above all, it's enormously enjoyable!

2 **apples** (Royal Gala or Golden Delicious)
1 small **parsnip** (unpeeled)
1 small handful fresh **mint**
1 small handful crushed **ice**

Place the apples, parsnip and mint into the juicer. Juice – pour over the ice – enjoy!

Juicy benefits Parsnips are part of the carrot family and, as is the case with most slow-growing root vegetables, parsnips are high in nutrients. They are packed with potassium and can therefore help reduce blood pressure. As with most fruit and vegetables, much of the flavour and goodness is found just beneath the skin, so it is important not to remove the skin before juicing.

little red roots

Mother Earth's finest beetroot, parsnip, carrot and radish juice

There is a theory that slow-growing root vegetables are high in nutrients as they absorb the goodness in the soil over a long period of time. This juice is vibrant red in colour and is literally plucked direct from Mother Earth herself.

½ **beetroot** (raw)
2 small **parsnips** (unpeeled)
2 **carrots**
1 **radish**
1 small handful crushed **ice**

Place the beetroot, parsnips, carrots and radish into the juicer. Juice – pour over ice – enjoy!

Juicy benefits Carrots and parsnips are from the same family and are an excellent source of potassium and magnesium. Carrot juice is renowned for its ability to cleanse the liver and it also has a particularly high level of beta-carotene (the anti-cancer king). It's worth mentioning that when you simply eat a carrot, your body can only assimilate about 1 per cent of the available beta-carotene, but when you juice it your body can assimilate nearly 100 per cent! Radishes have antibacterial properties and beetroot is also very useful for fighting off infections. This juice is superb for cleansing the liver, kidneys and bloodstream and is an excellent blood builder.

tomato twist

Vine-ripened **tomato** juice served on the rocks with a **twist** of **lemon**

Tomato juice is the real Marmite of the juice world, but whether you love or hate the taste, the benefits are undeniable.

6 **tomatoes**
⅓ **lemon** (peeled)
1 small handful crushed **ice**

Place the tomatoes and lime into the juicer. Juice – pour over the ice – enjoy!

Juicy benefits The healthy good looks of a fresh, red, ripe tomato are not just skin deep. Tomatoes are packed with health-promoting vitamins and disease-fighting phytonutrients, in particular the carotenoid lycopene. Lycopene is what gives the tomato its bright red colour and it has enormous significance in disease prevention. Lycopene is the most abundant carotenoid found in our blood and in an overwhelming number of studies tomatoes have been found to be invaluable in the fight against cancer.

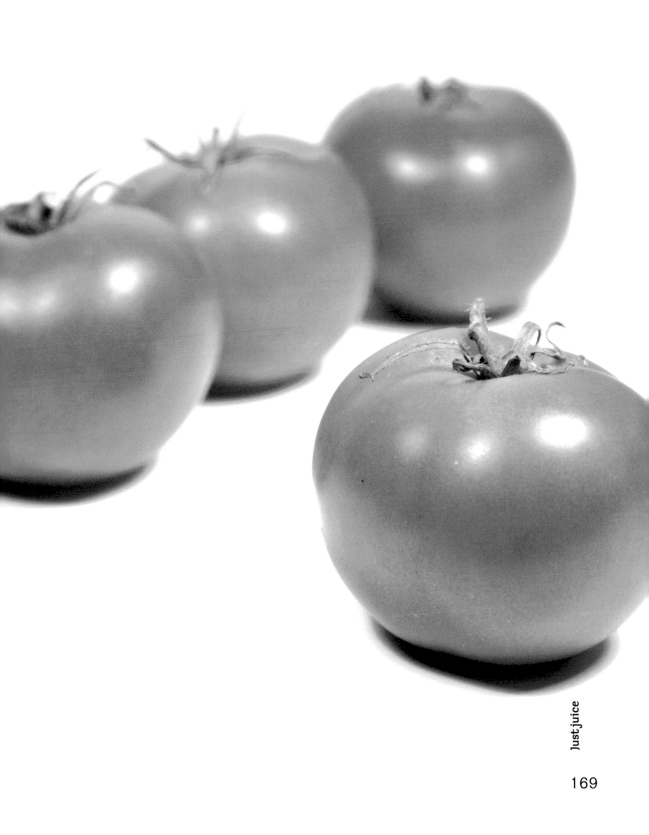

a little bit naughty…

Q: 'If we eat nothing but good food all our lives, do we live longer?'

A: 'No, but it sure feels like it!'

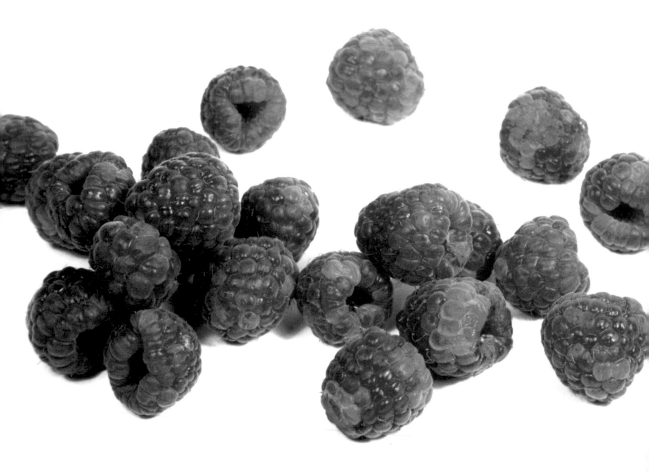

No matter who you are or how good your diet is, every now and then all of us just think 'sod it'! The recipes in this section are designed to meet your 'sod it' needs, but in a much more healthy and ethical way.

Ice cream, honey and even chocolate (!) are to be found in the following array of sweet smoothie delights. Who said healthy can't also be gorgeous …

Enjoy!

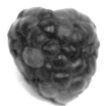

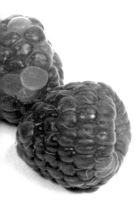

super naughty smoothie

Fresh blueberries, banana, pineapple juice, vanilla ice cream and a touch of Agave nectar

Some of the juices and smoothies in this section are slightly naughty, but whichever way you look at it, this one is super naughty (well, super naughty for this book anyway). It is the only smoothie in the book which contains ice cream, and I sense even the healthiest of you out there will be glad I have included it. However, as per all the recipes I do, there is always a health twist to it. Even though this has some cool delicious ice cream, this smoothie also contains an amazing quantity of vitamins, minerals and anti-oxidants. Not one to have all the time, but, hey, the body can easily handle a little of almost anything – enjoy!

1 **apple**
¼ medium **pineapple**
2 scoops **vanilla ice cream** (look for one which has little sugar in. Get real ice cream – maybe even organic)
½ **banana**
1 handful **blueberries**
1 teaspoon **Agave nectar** (an organic natural sweetener, it can be purchased in many supermarkets)
4 **ice** cubes

Juice the apple and pineapple and put into the blender along with the ice cream, the banana, blueberries, a squeeze of Agave nectar and ice. Blend all until smooth – flipping gorgeous! You may need a spoon. This makes enough for two, or one if you're feeling particularly naughty.

Look what's in it! Vitamins A, B1, B2 and B6, beta-carotene, calcium, iron, magnesium, phosphorus, sulphur, bromeline, folic acid, fibre, anti-oxidants, natural sugar (and, to be fair, unnatural sugars, depending on the ice cream you buy) and natural organically grown sweetener.

How will it juice me? First, it will taste so delicious that it will lift your spirits and, secondly, despite the ice cream, it will do a great deal of good internally. The bromeline contained in the pineapple encourages the secretion of hydrochloric acid, which will help to digest any of the protein in the ice cream. The many anti-oxidants help to destroy free radicals, and phosphorus is important as a building block for various carbohydrates and fats. Not bad for an apparently super naughty smoothie.

oh so sweet!

Freshly extracted orange juice, fresh kiwi fruit, and whole banana, all blended with Manuka active honey

Like most in this 'a bit naughty ... but nice' section, this recipe is, as it states, Oh So Sweet. However, like all the recipes, it is also Oh So Good For You!

Fruit smoothies are fantastic, but too much of even natural sugars can be a burden to your system. Always remember to drink slowly – after all, you would never swallow one whole banana and a kiwi fruit in one go. Allow the saliva in your mouth to do its work before swallowing. Enjoy your drink, don't just gulp it down.

2 large **oranges** (peeled but leave on white pith)
1 **banana** (fairtrade if you can – peeled)
1 **kiwi** fruit (peeled)
1 teaspoon **Manuka active honey**
ice cubes

Simply juice the oranges and place into the blender along with the banana, kiwi fruit, honey and ice – blend the lot until smooth.

Look what's in it! Vitamins A, B6, C and E, calcium, magnesium, potassium, fibre, beta-carotene, folic acid, iron, thiamine, natural sugars, amino acids and the antibacterial properties of the Manuka active honey.

How will it juice me? Manuka active honey is specially sourced from pollution-free areas of New Zealand. It is perhaps the most natural sweetener in the world and the 'active' properties mean that it is extremely antibacterial. This natural sugar, along with the natural sugars in the fruits, will give your system a natural juice high. The calcium is excellent for neutralizing any excess acid in the body, and the many, many vitamins, minerals and anti-oxidants will help to feed and protect every cell in your body.

> I started juicing a while back as I bought a juicer and one of Jason's book. I have always tried to watch what I eat but reading the book was very helpful in getting me to juice every evening after work. I have had people amazed when they taste how good the juices can be. it's now part of my life and everyone is telling me how good I look.

Marianne

dreamy strawberry delight

Fresh whole **strawberries**, freshly extracted **pineapple** juice and low-fat live **yogurt**

Dreamy is such an apt name for this rich and creamy smoothie. It tastes like a strawberry milkshake, only it is really good for you (and the kids)! By rights, this smoothie shouldn't even be in the 'little bit naughty' section as it's not really naughty at all, but when you taste it, it does feel like you are being naughty. It is not only good for you, but with the 98 per cent fat-free yogurt – it's pretty light too.

½ medium **pineapple**
1 large handful fresh **strawberries**
200g low-fat live **yogurt**
4 **ice** cubes

Juice the pineapple and add to blender along with the strawberries, yogurt and ice. Blend all until smooth.

Look what's in it! Vitamins C and E, calcium, magnesium, potassium, fibre, phosphorus, sulphur, ellagic acid, beta-carotene, folic acid, iron, thiamine, sodium, natural sugars, amino acids and friendly bacteria.

How will it juice me? Strawberries are loaded with vitamin C and beta-carotene, along with calcium, sodium, potassium and iron. Strawberries are also one of the few fruits that contain natural painkillers, some of which form the basis of synthetic drugs such as aspirin. The sulphur protects against toxic substances and the calcium is not only excellent for the bones and teeth, but helps to neutralize any excess acid in the body.

i can't believe it's good for me!

This is one of those smoothies that, when you taste it, you will automatically think, 'I can't believe it's good for me!' The old adage of 'It tastes good so it can't be good for me' has gone out of the window. I think all of the juices and smoothies in this book taste from pretty damn good to amazing – even the veggie ones! But sometimes there is one that is like an angel dancing on your tastebuds. This smoothie is soooooooo sweet that it will take an open and educated mind to accept it's all good.

¼ medium **pineapple**
2 **peaches** (de-stoned)
2 tablespoons low-fat live **yogurt**
A good squeeze of **Agave nectar**
Crushed **ice**

Simply juice the peaches and pineapple and place into the blender, along with the crushed ice, yogurt and a big squeeze of Agave nectar. Blend until smooth – soooooooooooooooooo nice!

Look what's in it! Vitamins A, B3 and C, beta-carotene, flavonoids, potassium, iron, anti-oxidants, folic acid, natural sugars, amino acids, natural fatsa and friendly bacteria.

How will it juice me? Peaches are one of nature's beta-carotene kings and as such are excellent for the prevention of many ailments, including cancer. They are very alkalizing and cleansing to the intestinal tract, encourage good bowel movement and help to clean the bladder and kidneys. This smoothie also helps to replenish the good bacteria in the gut, is very filling and – yes – it's good for you!

A little bit naughty

177

Juicy Fruit Facts

Fruit	Vitamins	Minerals	Juicy extras	Juice or smoothie?	Good for ...
Apple	A, B1, B2, B6, C	calcium, chlorine, magnesium, phosphorus, potassium, sulphur, iron	malic acid, nectin, ellagic acid	juice – but can be used for fruit or vegetable smoothies; can also be blended to add thickness and fibre to a smoothie	anti-cancer health promoter; pectin forms a gel in the intestine that eliminates toxins
Apricot	B, C, beta-carotene	sodium, potassium, magnesium, iron, calcium, silicon, boron		smoothie	energy, stamina, endurance; excellent blood builder; helping with heart disease; promoting shiny hair, glowing skin
Banana	B, C, beta-carotene, folic acid	potassium, magnesium, calcium, sodium		smoothie **Warning – bananas do not juice!**	slow release energy; immune booster; staving off symptoms of PMS; helping lower cholestrol
Blueberry	B1, B2, B6, C, beta-carotene, folic acid	calcium, iron, magnesium, manganese, phosphorus, potassium, sodium, zinc	ellagic acid	smoothie	slowing down the signs of ageing; destroying free radicals
Blackcurrant	C, beta-carotene	potassium, calcium, magnesium, phosphorus,		smoothie – makes a wonderful, but expensive juice	anti-cancer heath promoter; anti-bacterial; immune enhancer

Fruit	Vitamins	Minerals	Juicy extras	Juice or smoothie?	Good for ...
Cherry	B, C, beta-carotene	calcium, magnesium, zinc, iron, phosphorus, potassium, sulphur, copper, silicon	pectin, ellagic acid	smoothie – but makes a wonderful, but expensive juice	anti-cancer health promoter; controlling blood cholesterol levels and pectin also forms a gel in the intestine that eliminates toxins
Cranberry	B, C, beta-carotene, folic acid	iodine, calcium, chlorine, magnesium, phosphorus, potassium	quinine	juice or smoothie	Helping with liver, kidney, prostate or bladder problems
Grapefruit	C, beta-carotene	calcium, potassium	salicylic acid, pectin	juice	breaking down and shifting inorganic calcium from the joints; great at stimulating digestion
Grape	B, C, E, beta-carotene	iron, calcium, phosphorus, potassium	pectin	juice	helping to calm the nervous system; promoting good bowel movement; cleansing the system; restoring alkaline balance

Fruit	Vitamins	Minerals	Juicy extras	Juice or smoothie?	Good for ...
Kiwi	C, E, beta-carotene	calcium, magnesium, phosphorus, potassium, sodium		juice or smoothie	cleansing and energizing
Lemon/Lime	C, beta-carotene	calcium, magnesium, phosphorus, potassium	bioflavonoids, citric acid	juice (add a small amount to other fruit or vegetable juices)	cleansing the system – the acid scours the intestinal tract; eliminating toxins; neutralizing harmful bacteria
Mango	B, C, beta-carotene	calcium, copper, magnesium, phosphorus, iron		smoothie	mopping up free radicals; internal body cleanser; stimulating the immune system; disinfecting the body and reducing body odour
Melon	A, C, folic acid	calcium, zinc, potassium, magnesium, phosphorus		juice (using the entire fruit)	cooling the body; cleansing the kidneys; purifying the skin; promoting shiny hair, strong nails

Fruit	Vitamins	Minerals	Juicy extras	Juice or smoothie?	Good for ...
Nectarine	B1, B2, B3, B5, B6, C, beta-carotene, folic acid	calcium, magnesium, zinc, iron, phosphorus, potassium, copper		smoothie – but makes a wonderful, but expensive juice	anti-cancer health promoter and natural energizer
Orange	A, B6, C, beta-carotene, folic acid	calcium, iron, potassium, phosphorus, zinc	citric acid	juice (leaving pith on)	destroying free radicals that cause signs of skin ageing; scouring the intestine and flushing toxins from the body
Papaya	C, beta-carotene	calcium, magnesium	protedytic enzymes	smoothie	enabling easy digestion of complex proteins; promotes male fertility
Peach	B3, C, beta-carotene, folic acid	calcium, magnesium, zinc, iron, phosphorus, potassium, sulphur, copper, silicon		smoothie – but makes a wonderful, but expensive juice	fighting disease; anti-cancer health promoter; cleansing the intestine, bladder and kidneys

Fruit	Vitamins	Minerals	Juicy extras	Juice or smoothie?	Good for …
Pear	B6, C	copper, potassium		juice	controlling diabetes: contains levulose — a fruit sugar more easily tolerated by people with diabetes
Pineapple	B, C, E, folic acid	potassium, iron, calcium, sodium, phosphorus	bromeline	juice — but can be used for fruit or vegetable smoothies; can also be blended to add thickness and fibre to a smoothie	bromeline is an enzyme that aids digestion and helps dissolve excess mucus so is useful for hay fever and asthma
Raspberry	B, C, E, beta-carotene, niacin	calcium, iron, potassium, magnesium, phosphorus, sodium, zinc	ellagic acid	smoothie	maintaining healthy male reproductive function; promoting healthy skin; slowing down the signs of ageing
Strawberry	B, C, E, beta-carotene, folic acid, niacin	calcium, potassium, iron, sodium, magnesium, phosphorus, sulphur, zinc	ellagic acid	smoothie — but makes a wonderful, but expensive juice	building blood; boosting the immune system; slowing down the signs of ageing

Juicy Vegetable Facts

Vegetable	Vitamins	Minerals	Juicy extras	Juice or smoothie?	Good for ...
Avocado	B, C, beta-carotene	potassium, calcium, iron, phosphorus	essential natural fats	smoothie **Warning – do not juice avocado!**	a balanced diet: contains all 6 human nutritional needs in abundance – water, fat, protein, natural sugar, vitamins and minerals
Beetroot	B, C, beta-carotene, folic acid	chlorine, manganese, calcium, iron, sodium, phosphorus, potassium, chromium, magnesium	although a veg, tastes sweet	juice	cleansing the liver; iron deficiency anaemia; helping reduce hardening and blockage of the arteries
Broccoli	B, C, beta-carotene, folic acid	calcium, iron, phosphorus, potassium, sulphur		juice	high blood pressure; liver problems; constipation
Carrot	B, C, D, E, K, beta-carotene	calcium, iron, phosphorus, potassium, sulphur, chromium, magnesium, sodium, iodine, silica	although a veg, tastes sweet	juice	promoting healthy eyes; skin problems; cleansing the liver

Vegetable	Vitamins	Minerals	Juicy extras	Juice or smoothie?	Good for ...
Celery	B, C	calcium, iron, phosphorus, potassium, sulphur, sodium		juice	reducing acidity, so useful for arthritis and gout; natural diuretic; reducing fluid retention; calming the nervous system
Cucumber	B, C, beta-carotene	sodium, silica, manganese, sulphur, potassium, calcium, phosphorus, chlorine, magnesium		juice	excellent diuretic; reducing fluid retention; superb for the hair, nails and skin; helping reduce blood pressure
Fennel	B, C, beta-carotene	calcium, chromium, cobalt, iron, magnesium, manganese, phosphorus, potassium, selenium, silicon, sodium, zinc		juice	reducing intestinal gas, flatulence and bloating; calming effect on digestion
Ginger	C	copper, potassium, sodium, iron, calcium, zinc, phosphorus, magnesium		juice	natural antibiotic and decongestant

Vegetable	Vitamins	Minerals	Juicy extras	Juice or smoothie?	Good for ...
Parsnip	C, K, folic acid	potassium, iron, calcium, manganese		juice	helping to reduce blood pressure
Peppers	B, C, beta-carotene, folic acid	potassium, silica, iron, calcium, phosphorus, magnesium		juice	cleansing liver and intestine
Spinach	B, C, K, beta-carotene, folic acid	iron, iodine, calcium, phosphorus, potassium, sulphur		juice	anaemia – supporting effective liver and kidney function
Tomato	B, C, K	potassium, calcium, iron, phosphorus, iodine	lycopene	juice or smoothie	helpful for high blood pressure; cleansing the liver; lycopene has renowned anti-cancer properties
Watercress	B, C, E, beta-carotene, folic acid	sulphur, calcium, iron, sodium, magnesium, phosphorus, chlorine, potassium, iodine		juice	cleansing the liver; reducing fluid retention; healthy kidney function

index

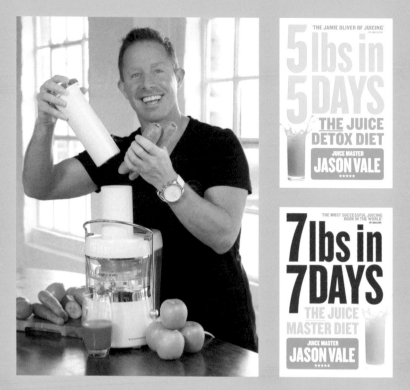

Jason Vale has been described as one of the leading authorities on health, addiction and juicing.

After turning his own life around with the help of a freshly-extracted juice programme, he set out on a mission to 'Juice the World'; he has spent the last 15 years spreading his message to people from every corner of the globe. His books have now sold over 3 million copies and been translated into many languages.

For more information on the Juice Booster range, Juice Master books, CDs, DVDs, forthcoming seminars, juice-bar opportunities, plus anything else you need to know about our juicy world, please contact us at:

Website: **www.juicemaster.com**
Email: **info@juicemaster.com**